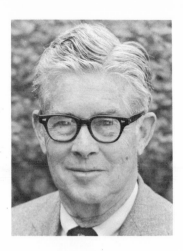

FREDRICK J. STARE

Fredrick J. Stare, M.D., Ph.D., is Professor Emeritus and founder of Harvard University's Department of Nutrition. He is also co-founder and Chairman, Board of Directors, of the American Council on Science and Health.

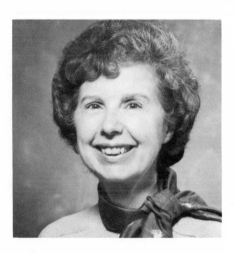

MARGARET MCWILLIAMS

Margaret McWilliams, R.D., Ph.D., is a professor of food and nutrition at California State University in Los Angeles, where she served as chairman of the home economics department for eight years. She received her Ph.D. in food and nutrition from Oregon State University. The author or co-author of ten texts on nutrition, Dr. McWilliams is now Coordinator of Health-Related Programs and Program Director of the Coordinated Undergraduate Dietetics Program at California State.

Nutrition for Good Health

Second Edition

Eating less and living longer!

by
Fredrick J. Stare, M.D., Ph.D.
    Professor and Founder
    Department of Nutrition
    Harvard University

Margaret McWilliams, Ph.D., R.D.
    Professor of Food and Nutrition
    Department of Home Economics
    California State University, Los Angeles

George F. Stickley Company   210 West Washington Square
Philadelphia, PA 19106

Manufactured in the United States of America; Published by the
George F. Stickley Company, 210 W. Washington Square,
Philadelphia, PA. 19106.

FOREWORD

Throughout history, and probably before, mankind has always been fascinated by diet and nutrition. The Hippocratic writings, almost a thousand years before Christ, are full of advice about the cure and prevention of disease by diet, but the current popular clamor on the subject is unmatched in history. Instinctively we tend to accept the dictum of Brillat-Savarin, who wrote, "Tell me what you eat and I'll tell you what you are," and of Goethe's famous play on German words, meaning in English, "Man is what he eats."

The more recent development of the science of nutrition has given enormous detail to the older wisdom and therein is the source of the confusion and outlandish claims that beset us today. For the metabolism of the nutrients is so complicated, and still so replete with uncertainty at the cellular level, that nonsense is easily built out of half truth and imagination garnished with some pseudoscientific jargon. So we have the diet of the month, the succession of claims about how to gain health and vigor and lose weight without effort by following the latest dietary "breakthrough."

Actually, as this book shows, the practical fundamentals of nutrition are not difficult to understand nor is it necessary to be a biochemist to assure that your diet meets all your needs. To be sure, in some illnesses and rare metabolic disorders a medical specialist may be required but for the vast majority of people "Nutrition for Good Health" gives all the answers. It is easy to understand, well-balanced, and up-to-the-minute.

Aside from the continuing commercial exploitation of unnecessary vitamin and mineral preparations, the current popular dietary interests in the United States concern how to reduce, fats in the diet, and fiber. On reducing, there is no escaping the fact that calorie intake and calorie expenditure determine the outcome. On dietary fats, the American diet is commonly too rich in fats, especially the saturated fats of animal origin, but this fault is easily corrected. Fiber in the diet, long dismissed as merely undigestible "filler," is a new commercial enthusiasm; foods are processed to get rid of fiber and then, with much fanfare, fiber (bran) is added to the packaged food. All these matters are explained simply in "Nutrition for Good Health."

Ancel Keys, Ph.D., *Professor Emeritus, Laboratory of Physiological Hygiene, University of Minnesota*

PREFACE

As we have worked in the field of nutrition over the years, we have grown increasingly aware of the need for understandable and accurate nutrition information for consumers. This book is written to provide the answers to nutrition questions that presently are being asked by the public. This is the revised edition of the second book in which the two authors, one on the East Coast and the other on the West Coast, have collaborated. It results from the success of the first collaborative effort which was a college and university textbook titled "Living Nutrition" published by John Wiley and Sons, New York. "Living Nutrition" is now in its third edition.

"Nutrition for Good Health" can be viewed as a type of nutrition supplement for you. We have attempted to identify the most pressing questions you may have about what to eat to be well nourished in this complex scene in which we all live. Our discussions are presented in practical terms for today's busy consumers. The book is designed so that you can read short segments on questions you may have. It can be read from "cover to cover" or in any order you choose. Each topic is presented independently and does not rely on previous chapters for interpretation. You can enjoy the short articles as a bedside reader or as entertainment for a rainy day.

We hope this book provides you with the information you have been seeking about your diet. Nutrition is truly a vital science for all of us.

March, 1982

FREDRICK J. STARE
MARGARET MCWILLIAMS

CONTENTS

WEIGHTY MATTERS

It's a pretty safe bet that the subject of weight control and diets will be discussed at some time during the course of virtually any social event these days. Americans are worried about their weight because of the effects of obesity on health and longevity as well as on appearance. It may indeed be a matter of life and death. Clearly, this matter of controlling weight is one of the nation's vital nutritional concerns.

Life in the United States today seems to be one of contradictions. On one hand we are bombarded with sales pitches for many delectable foods, while countless solutions to overeating—some on the wild side and some conservative—can be found at any time in popular magazines, books, and other media reaching the lay public. Advice on weight loss certainly is not hard to find. The challenge is to find a safe solution that works for you and that *maintains* your weight at the desired level!

To start things off, let's look at some of the questions about obesity. Some of the answers are far from easy; in fact they are not yet solved. But there are facts we do know, and these are of great interest because two in every five persons in the United States is fat—and getting fatter.

Is obesity really a hazard, or is this just a matter of opinion, custom, and taste?

The most important fact is that obesity is a hazard, particularly when it is combined with other health hazards such as cigarette smoking, elevated blood pressure, physical inactivity, etc. A fat person is seldom just fat, but often has other health hazards or diseases. Studies and figures by experts in medicine and in insurance all agree that extra fat is a complication in heart disease, diabetes, other disorders, and surgery. By and large, obesity is risky. Slimness is not just a matter of style—it is also important to survival!

Do calories count, or do you gain weight if it is your nature?

Emphatically, calories *do* count. The body uses calories for basal metabolism (basic survival), activity, and the processing of the food we eat. It obtains these calories from three sources: food, drink, and body fat. Weight remains relatively constant when the calories consumed daily from food and drink regularly equal the total calories expended. On the other hand, if there is a deficit of calories, either from eating and drinking less or from using more (as a result of exercise), the body turns to its own fat and burns this for fuel to make up the deficit. The result is just what the dieter is seeking—weight is lost. When there are more calories consumed than are needed, the excess is stored in the body as fat (much to the dismay of the dieter).

We do not know all the reasons why some people eat and drink too much, but we do know that no diet is successful if it supplies too many calories. Any diet results in weight loss as long as it cuts down on calories to the point where the food eaten does not supply as many calories as the energy needed by the body. And when we include "drink" along with food as a source of calories, we are talking about alcoholic beverages and soft drinks.

Unfortunately, simply cutting down on calories is not the answer. To be effective, a diet must include all the essential nutrients, and it must take into consideration an individual's likes and dislikes. A diet must not be punishing, and it cannot be magical. Fast weight loss by rigid restriction is poor practice, for the pounds soon pile up again. The only way to win the battle of the bulge is to beat a slow and steady retreat. This will help to make the reduction a lasting one, for habits can be changed slowly and permanently.

Does exercise help weight loss, or does it work the other way by increasing the appetite?

Exercise will help. For many, it is more important than diet. Moderate and regular exercise does not increase the appetite, and it does burn up extra calories. For example, two brisk 15-minute walks every day for a year can remove 15 pounds—far better, certainly, than adding 15 pounds! As a fringe benefit, exercise improves the circulation, increases muscle tone, lessens tensions and anxieties, makes you feel better, and increases the general feeling of well being.

How much weight is too much?

This is a personal problem to be determined by you and your doctor.

A BUDGET OF A DIFFERENT KIND

Budgeting is essential, whether you are dealing with dollars and cents or with food and sense. In the case of weight control, calories and exercise are the coins of the realm. Exercise alone seldom reduces weight. You also have to be wise about what you eat.

Just as you can't pay for a new coat with the contents of a piggy bank, neither can you pay, calorically, for a long, cold alcoholic beverage with a few swings of a golf club. Nor will that bag of peanuts be burned up while you climb to your seat at the ball game, even if it is the highest, hottest seat in all of the bleachers. So if you want your accounts to balance, you may need to exercise more and eat less, including drinking fewer alcoholic beverages. Balanced budgeting of all kinds can only be achieved if there is a balance between what you put in and what you put out.

If you are among the more than 50 percent of Americans who are overweight, you'll want to think about establishing a brand new set of habits of physical activity and eating, a set that will help you gain and maintain the weight needed for optimal health. Moderation is the key to dieting and weight control. That means that you need to eat a wide array of foods every day, but less of everything.

Don't be tempted with one of the many fad diets that you have seen advertised. They inevitably lead to the ceaseless process of losing and gaining, which can be discouraging, dangerous, and as useless as trying to eliminate weeds by cutting off their tops. To remove the roots of the problem, it is necessary to set up a new plan of regular physical activity and eating designed to last a lifetime.

Here are some guidelines for reducing that you may find helpful:

1. Adjust servings to meet your own needs. Some people find it helpful to have a portion of lunch or dinner before the regular meal to reduce the appetite. But remember when you do this that you have eaten part of that meal in advance. The amount of food on your plate at the actual meal must be minus the food already eaten.
2. Calories in snacks can mount up quickly. If you are famished for a snack during the middle of the morning or afternoon, select a snack that is low in calories, such as coffee, tea, bouillon, pickles, raw vegetables, or small portions of raw fruits.
3. Add zest to meals with non-caloric spices and herbs, and go easy with butter, margarine, and salt.
4. Use flour, cornstarch, sugar, honey, syrup, and other sweets sparingly. Avoid fruit canned with sugar syrups.
5. Reduce fats by such devices as trimming fat from meats and avoiding dishes containing large amounts of butter or other fat, including fried and fatty foods, nuts, hot rolls with butter, biscuits, sauces, gravies, salad dressings, pastries, and desserts. While all these foods may be consumed, the portions should be small. The secret is cutting down, not out!

6. All beverages and drinks, hard and soft, must be counted among the total day's calories. The only exceptions are water, low-calorie soft drinks, and tea and coffee without added sugar or cream.
7. Chew slowly, enjoy your food, and thus gain time to achieve that satisfied feeling which eliminates the need for second helpings.
8. Plan to eat with regularity as much as possible. Skipping meals is a poor practice, for it usually leads to fatigue, excessive nibbling, overeating, and haphazard nutrition.
9. Recognize a "normal" portion size. The size of a hamburger, steak, or baked potato served in a restaurant should not necessarily be your standard. Three ounces of cooked meat, an amount usually far less than the serving in a restaurant, is really all you need to provide the protein for a meal.
10. Keep weekly (not daily) tabs on your progress with a scale and a tape measure. Do not reach for the moon. It will take a while for you to begin to move out from the launch (or is it the lunch?) pad. Weight loss by rigid restriction may be spectacular, but it seldom is lasting, and it may be dangerous to your health. Gradual weight loss is far more effective and more apt to be lasting.

Individuals can lose weight and be greatly benefited without the need for rigid self-denial of enjoyable eating. Be careful not to eliminate any one group of foods from your dieting plan. Each group is essential to good health, and that includes the bread and cereal group which so many dieters condemn and abandon. Every day you will need a variety of low-calorie, nutrient-dense foods selected from the Basic Four Food Groups: fruits and vegetables; milk and cheese; cereals and breads; and meats, poultry, fish, and eggs.

Along with your "less-is-best" diet plan, set up regular habits of exercise, whether that means a brisk daily walk, a couple of sets of tennis, golf (without a golf cart), gardening, jumping rope, or even playing racquetball. Exercise that produces a little huffing and puffing is good for most people. It helps the circulation and it certainly aids in burning up the calories.

But don't forget that budget. After exercising, if you want to lose weight, have a nice cold glass of water instead of one of those tempting hard or soft drinks.

THE TONIC SCALE

The best beginning is by making exercise a do-it-yourself program. Fat does not boil off with steam baths, nor does it rub off with massage. Fat is stored energy, and it has to be burned off by regular physical effort—your own effort.

Weekend sports, like crash diets, are not very helpful in weight reduction. The muscles you move, the pounds you lose on a vigorous weekend or a quick-cure diet build up your hopes, but they do not do much to permanently diminish your waistline. This kind of loss is strictly temporary. It lasts only until the excitement dies down and you return to your usual routines. You have not accomplished a permanent change and, what is more, you may have done damage. The off-again, on-again program can be more harmful to you than overweight itself.

The only constructive long-term solution is regular moderate exercise, day by day, week in and week out, year after year. Such a physical conditioning program is good because it does not increase appetite, and it does not cause one to eat more. Furthermore, it is the best way to figure control and weight loss without flabbiness. Here are some figures to think about in relation to yours:

Type of exercise	Calories used in ½-hour
Sitting	45
Standing	60
Walking	110
Golfing	150
Tennis (singles)	250
Swimming or rowing	250

Then remember that there are 60 calories in a slice of bread, 75 in a potato, 120 in a glass of beer, 140 in a highball, and almost 400 in a piece of pie, a sundae, or a quarter-pound serving of meat. It's a simple matter of arithmetic.

A PRACTICAL PHILOSOPHY

The secret to success in weight control is to eat well, but with wisdom and restraint. One fact is certain—you won't be fat if you eat only what you need. The one sure way to lose weight is to keep your calories in line with your requirements. All reducing diets rely on the same method. Basically, they limit your caloric intake, no matter how alluring the ads and the fads, no matter what they promise and proclaim.

A calorie measures the amount of energy a food supplies to the body. When the diet is based on an intake that provides less energy than the body needs, weight will be lost. This is the basis of weight reduction diets. The total intake of calories from all foods and beverages must be controlled if weight is to be lost. Regardless of their sources (solid food or liquid, meat or potato, fat or sugar, soft drink or hard), too many calories today, tomorrow, and the next day will make you fat.

Our machine age has made it all too easy to avoid exercise and activity. Today we sit instead of stand, ride instead of walk, and flip switches instead of flexing muscles. At work we push buttons and pencils, while at rest we sit and watch television. To compound the problem, we nibble while we look. In essence, we are living in the era of machine power while hanging onto the food habits of the days of man power. Fortunately, the current fitness movement is helping to modify this picture and to firm the figures of those who are participating.

Sometimes there are other reasons for obesity. Unhappiness is a cause of indulgence. All too often eating is an outlet for emotions during periods of stress or boredom, and then a lasting habit of overeating is established. The overweight which results interferes with normal job performance and social life, and this in turn leads to more overeating as a solace for the misery. Seldom do glandular disturbances cause obesity, despite the convenience of claiming this problem as the culprit.

By and large, your weight is up to you, and control is up to you. Dieting is hard work, as anyone who has tried it will tell you. But the hard work will pay off immeasurably in the way you look and feel once you have shed the surplus pounds and found yourself to be the trim person you always wanted to be.

TRAPPING YOUR WEIGHT PROBLEM

Do you find that your intentions to diet are exciting and promising, but that they fall by the wayside as you encounter various traps? Many pitfalls confront the dieter, but here are some ideas for coping with them.

The loaded refrigerator and cupboards groaning with the burden you have just stowed in them when you returned from the grocery store can be a real threat to any diet. This often is your first day of danger because everything looks so tempting and smells so good. Besides, you may be a bit tired and hungry after shopping so hard! It is pretty easy under these circumstances to decide that you deserve just a bit of a reward for doing such good deeds.

That's when you will need to remind yourself emphatically that the coffee cake is for the children, and the celery, carrots, and cottage cheese are for you. This is a good time to depart quickly from the kitchen and take up some other activity. You may even be able to convince yourself that you really don't want any of that coffee cake. And certainly you would prefer to see one pound less on the scale, rather than one pound more, the next time you weigh yourself.

And could you possibly define yourself as a "night crawler," that stealthy dieter who believes that food eaten when others sleep doesn't really count? Are you suddenly thirsty and so hungry in the middle of the night that you can't get back to sleep without a snack?

Perhaps you're on your way to get a glass of water when you suddenly discover that you really are hungry or need just a little food to settle the stomach—maybe a piece of cold fried chicken beckons. Don't fool yourself that you can eat while others sleep without paying the penalty. The scale will creep slowly upward as these midnight forays escalate.

If you are a regular member of the night patrol, the first step to curing this problem is the declaration that the kitchen is off-limits to yourself. This may be easier to enforce if you don't even let yourself get out of bed. You can accomplish this by solving your thirst problem and keeping a glass of water right beside the bed so you can reach it without getting up or turning on the light.

Next, try some deep breathing exercises while also concentrating on what it will feel like to slim down to fit clothes that are the next size smaller. Then close your eyes and relax. Begin methodically with your toes and work upward to relax every muscle, being sure to give special attention to relaxing the face muscles, including the eyebrows.

If you are still awake, imagine the weight, pound by pound, leaving your body; think how nice it will feel to be free of the burden of carrying such a heavy load with you whenever you move. Remember, too, that you have to brush your teeth again if you nibble at night, a requirement you can impose on yourself to help avoid night snacks.

Are you the Chairman of the "Bored"? Boredom can be the cause of obesity, for eating often is viewed as a very pleasant diversion in the middle of nothing to do. Distractions are in order to prevent the practice of eating just for something to do. Make a list of the sundry tasks you have been putting off for eons. Each time you begin to feel bored, keep yourself occupied by doing something from that list. Productive tasks are far more rewarding than eating a candy bar which will simply compound the weight problem. Tackle the mending, clean a closet, straighten your desk, do your nails, or do anything, but work toward a feeling of accomplishment. Then pick up the phone and call someone who is fun to talk with. Once you are occupied, your boredom will disappear faster than a bowl of peanuts.

Solicitous friends can also pose problems for the dieter. You may need to find ways to outwit friends who urge you to eat with some innocent comments, such as, "Oh, just one taste won't hurt." It is truly amazing how many people rather thoughtlessly make it difficult for you to stay on your diet. However, you can avoid their urging by having some answers ready. You can say that you would rather talk than eat, that you really aren't hungry, that you just ate, or even that you've developed a new allergy. Whatever you do, don't mention the word "diet." If you do, your friends may be convinced that you are starving yourself and really pressure you to eat. Your best defense is to think of a new subject to talk about immediately.

Avoid food rewards for "good behavior" while on a diet. You may need to control your thoughts, to keep your feeling of success in your diet even when the scale seems to be plateauing for awhile. Remember, you are in charge of your own thoughts. When you are thinking of straying into such dangerous thoughts as cheating on your diet, concentrate on the lift you know you will get when you reach your desired slimmer silhouette. With such a thought, why would you allow yourself to cheat on the diet and delay the time when you can see the "new you" and enjoy the feeling of success? Why would you allow yourself to continue to be dragged down by excess weight when you can soon be enjoying the pleasures of a thinner you? Keep positive thoughts in your mind. When you are not weighed down with depressing, negative thoughts, you can rescue yourself from the realm of the obese!

DON'T LET YOUR FIGURE GO UP IN SMOKE

So you have actually decided that the statistics on the risks of smoking apply to you, and now that means that the task of breaking the smoking habit is about to begin. Before you begin, consider how you are going to avoid gaining weight. Start by recognizing that people may gain weight when they stop smoking because of a couple of important reasons: people who smoke are in the habit of putting something in their fingers and mouths that they enjoy, namely cigarettes. Without cigarettes, they want other things in their fingers and mouths, namely food—candies, gum, and snacks—and up go the calorie intake and the weight. Also, most people who stop smoking find that their food tastes better to them. Consequently, they down the food, and the weight goes up.

Here are some specific tips that have helped many people to avoid putting on weight while they are breaking the smoking habit. These ideas may help you avoid gain and may even result in a bit of weight loss. First, have something besides food to put in your fingers—a pencil or pen, perhaps, and even chew on the end, if necessary; omit all added salt from the food for the first couple of weeks. After that period, continue by using salt only in cooking and never at the table. Why? The food won't have the same taste appeal for you, and you will eat less than you would with more salt on the food. Take no second servings—ever; eat more frequently, but in smaller quantities. Have a snack in the mid-morning, mid-afternoon, and at bedtime. Just make sure that the snacks you eat would have been a part of the next meal and not just something extra. Get more exercise; a good brisk walk around the block before dinner and after dinner, plus a brisk noonday walk of about 15 minutes can be highly beneficial. This daily exercise (and it is important that it be almost daily) helps you burn up calories while also improving your health through improved circulation and better muscle tone.

Most smoking deterrents are pills or tablets consisting of nothing more than spices, flavorings such as licorice, cloves, ginger, and menthol. Lobelia (or lobeline sulfate) is an alkaloid drug which some people think is helpful in suppressing the desire to smoke. Group therapy similar to Alcoholics Anonymous may be helpful. There are many plans and aids available to help people stop smoking. An active and sustained determination to stop is essential, and the few tips given here will help you avoid unnecessary and undesirable weight gain when you do give it up. Good luck!

Now that we have looked at some general ways of working toward weight control, let's briefly reflect on the origin and continuity of the overweight problem in the United States.

BIRTH OF THE GIRTH

It will doubtless not come as any great surprise to you that overnutrition is probably the biggest nutrition problem in the United States today. By overnutrition, we mean simply that people are consuming more calories (from food and drink) than they need for good health, and this surplus consumption gradually leads to that nagging problem of overweight. There is no age group, income bracket, or occupational classification that is not afflicted with this problem. You will notice overweight individuals anywhere you go in our country or in other countries. There are many reasons why we tend to eat more than we really need, but very frequently the basic cause or causes can be traced back to influences during childhood.

In years back, when medical knowledge was considerably more limited than it is today, parents undoubtedly noticed that plump children were often healthier than very thin ones. The plump children did not develop tuberculosis, for example. It was the thin children who were prone to become ill. This led to the attitude of some parents of urging children to eat, eat, eat. Eat and enjoy it!

Solicitous coaxing to eat became a way of life as a health protection measure. Today this approach to feeding children is still found in many families, and it is laying the foundation for eating habits that will cause these children to be overweight as adults. With advances in medical science, there appears to be no value in having children a bit heavier than the recommended weight for their height. Indeed, there is growing concern with the health hazards of overweight. And research has shown that obesity or overweight is most difficult to correct in individuals who have been overweight since infancy, possibly because such individuals may actually have more fat cells. There is good reason to encourage good eating patterns from infancy and continuing throughout life to avoid the beginnings of excess weight.

It is a common axiom in American life that we should eat all the food prepared for a meal and not let it go to waste. Parents will frequently urge children at their tables to finish different items so the food will not go to waste. The trouble with this is that this excess food will still go to "waist," that is, *your* waist rather than to waste. For health reasons, it is distinctly better to serve leftovers at another meal rather than encourage people to eat more food than their bodies need. Hostesses who chronically have small amounts left over would do far better either to prepare less food or to become creative in the art of disguising and preparing leftovers. You can help yourself and your family by encouraging weight control all the time. Avoid making people feel that you will be personally offended if they don't eat second and third helpings of your favorite recipes. It is fine to enjoy good food, but it is a health hazard to let too much food go to w-a-i-s-t.

As you can see, it is important to have all members of the family maintain a desirable weight for their heights and ages. Do you have children or grandchildren? Of course, they always look beautiful to their families, but just how do they look to others?

CHILDREN AND THEIR WEIGHT

Are the children in your family too thin, just right, pleasingly plump, cherubically chubby, or are they just plain fat and getting fatter? Weight control is important for good health at all ages, but it is perhaps most crucial in childhood. The importance of weight control in childhood may surprise you, for we all beam indulgently at plump babies and young children and forgivingly say that this is only "baby fat," and they will soon run it off. Usually we hear the greatest concern being voiced about middleaged adults with too much fat, because they are the ones most likely to collapse suddenly from a heart attack. However, we are concerned about children because it often is the overweight children who become the overweight adults—with the greatest difficulty in reducing and keeping reduced. Frequently, plump children are headed for an entire lifetime of overweight or actual obesity. Statistics definitely have shown that excess weight (particularly when such other risk factors as high blood pressure, cigarette smoking, elevated cholesterol, and diabetes are present) is a hazard to good health. It is harder to measure, but probably just as true, that excess weight has also led to a good deal of unhappiness. Even if you feel that it is true that blondes have more fun, you probably would not agree that fat blondes have more fun.

Although it is a simple matter to agree that people need to begin to control their weight in childhood and continue this practice throughout their lives, it is quite another to actually manage this. Here are a couple of pointers to remember in any attempts to lose weight.

If you want to help your children or yourself lose weight, you should seek a doctor's supervision unless you only have about five pounds to lose. Working with your doctor should be a dietitian or a nutritionist who will aid you in selecting a diet that is nourishing yet can result in a gradual weight loss. A good reducing diet retrains your eating habits while you are losing weight. That way, it is a rather easy matter to continue eating in this new way when you get to the desired weight. With the crash diets that claim to take weight off extremely quickly, most people find that they rapidly regain the lost weight because they go right back to their old eating habits and lack of exercise which caused them to be too heavy in the first place. Crash diets, starvation diets, liquid diets, etc. do not change eating habits. It is a good idea to reduce your weight by eating normal, well-balanced meals, being sure to keep the servings smaller than you usually eat. You have to learn to live with less food, not without it! Smaller servings of meat are particularly important because of the comparatively high calorie content of meat. Also, start now to substitute nonfat milk for whole milk. Avoid taking second helpings and skip most desserts (except *fresh* fruits). Try to content yourself with a cup of black coffee or unsweetened tea rather than eating dessert.

For exercise, try putting your hands firmly against the edge of the table and pushing back rather than reaching for seconds. At our house, we call this exercise the "push backs," and it works very well when you need to lose some weight. Of course, long brisk walks and other forms of physical activity are also important.

Children and adults alike usually find it easier to control weight if they develop an active outside interest so that they have less time to eat and to think about food. "Huffing and puffing" activities are recommended strongly as one of the outside activities.

So far, we have been talking about overweight and obesity in general terms. Now it is time to see what it really means to have a weight problem.

WHAT SHAPE ARE YOU IN?

Here is a typical question from an interested reader. *Could you please tell me what I should weigh? I have a small frame, weigh 130 pounds, am 5'4" tall, and am 28 years old.*

The answer to this question and similar ones is taken from the table of Desirable Weights developed by the Metropolitan Life Insurance Company. Note that the tables are structured to include the variables of size of frame and sex. Check in the appropriate table to determine what your desirable weight range is.

DESIRABLE WEIGHTS FOR MEN AGE 25 AND OVER*

Height (In Shoes With 1" Heel)	Weight in Indoor Clothing (Pounds)		
	Small Frame	Medium Frame	Large Frame
5'2"	112–120	118–129	126–141
5'3"	115–123	121–133	129–144
5'4"	118–126	124–136	132–148
5'5"	121–129	127–139	135–152
5'6"	124–133	130–143	138–156
5'7"	128–137	134–147	142–161
5'8"	132–141	138–152	147–166
5'9"	136–145	142–156	151–170
5'10"	140–150	146–160	155–174
5'11"	144–154	150–165	159–179
6'0"	148–158	154–170	164–184
6'1"	152–162	158–175	168–189
6'2"	156–167	162–180	173–194
6'3"	160–171	167–185	178–199
6'4"	164–175	172–190	182–204

* For weights between ages 18 and 25, subtract one pound for each year under 25.

DESIRABLE WEIGHTS FOR WOMEN AGE 25 AND OVER*

Height (In Shoes With 2" Heel)	Weight in Indoor Clothing (Pounds)		
	Small Frame	Medium Frame	Large Frame
4'10"	92–98	96–107	104–119
4'11"	94–101	98–110	106–122
5'0"	96–104	101–113	109–125
5'1"	99–107	104–116	112–128
5'2"	102–110	107–119	115–131
5'3"	105–113	110–122	118–134
5'4"	108–116	113–126	121–138
5'5"	111–119	116–130	125–142
5'6"	114–123	120–135	129–146
5'7"	118–127	124–139	133–150
5'8"	122–131	128–143	137–154
5'9"	126–135	132–147	141–158
5'10"	130–140	136–151	145–163
5'11"	134–144	140–155	149–168
6'0"	138–148	144–159	153–173

* For weights between the ages of 18 and 25, subtract one pound for each year under 25.

Now, to answer our reader's question. Assuming her height is 5'4" without two-inch heels, it is necessary to add two inches for heels in the Desirable Weight chart; her Desirable Weight would be within the range of 114 to 123 pounds, the range for a small-framed woman. This reader obviously weighs a few pounds more than is desirable for optimum health. She has not yet reached the point where a nutritionist would say that she is actually "overweight." The term "overweight" is used to designate a person who weighs between 10 and 20 percent more than the desirable body weight. In our reader's case, she would not be called overweight until she weighed about 134 pounds. If she continued to gain weight and eventually gained so much weight that she weighed 20 percent more than was desirable, she would be called "obese" by the experts.

When you are calculating your own condition, keep in mind that the preferred circumstance is to weigh in about the middle of the appropriate range for your height and body build. Avoid shopping through the table until you find the body frame and height that match up with your weight!

If you have just a bit of a weight problem, you simply need to modify your eating, drinking, and exercise habits a little, and success will be yours. Unfortunately, some of our readers may be similar to the 33-year-old man who wrote that he was 5'7" tall, weighed 285 pounds, and wanted a recommendation for a place to help him with his weight problem. The answer for him and others like him is to obtain help through a hospital that has an overweight or obesity clinic. Most health departments of states or large cities have consulting nutritionists who frequently provide dietary advice throughout their districts. A number of private organizations have been formed in which groups of individuals meet weekly to receive group instruction on weight loss and to encourage each other. Your local or state health department should be able to advise you if there is such an organization in your community.

Any reducing program, particularly for one who is markedly overweight, should begin with a thorough physical examination by a physician. And from then on, it is a long and consistent program of eating less and using your muscles more. Don't forget that the reduced amount of food still must provide the many nutrients needed for good health.

WEIGHT LISTINGS

Dieting can be a lonely process, or it can be done by participating in a group. For some people, the support of other group members who are also trying to lose weight can be of great benefit. Some groups also have the benefit of presenting sound nutrition education programs at their weekly meetings. Groups which have gained nationwide prominence in reducing circles are TOPS, Weight Watchers, and Diet Workshop. Each of these programs has its own dietary approach, but the principles involved are similar. Since these groups are usually businesses, fees are charged.

TOPS (Take Off Pounds Sensibly), founded in 1952, is probably the oldest of the self-help groups. It offers no particular diet of its own, but presents a balanced image of the principles of good nutrition and recommends that individuals consult their own physicians for specific diets. "Weighing in" precedes the weekly meeting and is done in private, with the records being kept by the staff. Competition is keen, and various awards are presented as part of the social activities. Emphasis is always on pounds lost rather than on current weight. Men's and women's groups originally met separately, on the assumption that it lessened embarrassment and that the two sexes didn't understand each other's weight problems anyway. However, in recent years they have been meeting together. For a follow-up program, there is also KOPS (Keep Off Pounds Sensibly).

Weight Watchers is a much more commercial organization than TOPS and has a line of food products available in retail markets to augment the meetings they conduct for dieters. Their current nutritional program was developed under the guidance of Dr. W. Henry Sebrell, a well qualified nutritionist and physician. Recent versions of their nutritional plan provide for individual selection of food and drink, while still emphasizing meals that are low in calories and nutritionally well balanced. Diet Workshop also emphasizes balanced diets and exercise.

Behavior modification, with heavy emphasis on the self-help concept, is an important part of the program. Members weigh in at each meeting and are acclaimed for losses. At meetings one or more times a week, members participate in group discussions under the leadership of a trained "role model." Discussions focus on self-help by each individual as a part of the group. Personal eating problems are discussed and compared, and members quickly discover that their personal difficulties are not unique. From this perspective, they identify correct eating habits to cover a variety of situations. Dieters are advised how to deal with other family members, friends, the frequent temptations to indulge in "forbidden" foods, and situations such as eating out. Gradually, members accept their eating problems as a normal reaction to certain kinds of stress, both physical and psychological. Positive, reinforcing responses are used to overcome the tendency to react to such stresses by overeating.

The Weight Watchers staff feel that the informal setting adds immeasurably to social interaction. They also feel that the collection of fees not only allows them to provide more effective service, but also provides a definite motivation for a paying member to continue on the diet program. Weight Watchers believes that motivation is almost as necessary to dieting success as is a rigorously controlled diet. Emphasis is given continually to developing, strengthening, and maintaining motivation in every member. In fact, even after the weight goal has been reached, individuals are encouraged to continue attendance at weekly meetings to maintain the motivation needed for weight maintenance.

These and other self-help groups are available in many places throughout the country to provide moral support and encouragement to dieters who desire this type of assistance in pursuing their dietary objective and who can afford the fees. Although long-term success cannot be guaranteed by these groups (or any other support system), their general approach of a balanced diet with somewhat reduced total intake is certainly not harmful to your health. In fact, some people have found this to be a successful route to permanent weight reduction.

Now, let's take a look at some suggestions for ways to lose weight sensibly and gradually.

THE LADY'S FARE

Here is a suggested plan for the 53-year-old saleslady who requested a diet that would allow her to lose 15 pounds safely and as quickly as possible. A daily intake of 1,200 kilocalories is suggested for the first two weeks and then the intake is increased to 1,400 kilocalories per day until the desired 15 pounds have been lost.

"Kilocalories" may be a new term to some. The caloric content of foods and caloric expenditure of exercise is measured in kilocalories which are 1,000 times the energy value of the measurement used in physics termed a calorie and spelled with a small "c". When calorie is spelled with a capital C—Calorie—it refers to a kilocalorie. However, in common usage dealing with the caloric values of foods or exercise, the word is frequently spelled with a small "c", as we do in this book, even though we are referring to a kilocalorie or a Calorie.

A proposed menu for the day is:

Breakfast	Fruit or juice
	Cereal with skim milk (no sugar)
	or
	Poached egg plus one slice of toast
	Coffee
Lunch	Tomato consommé
	Cottage cheese and fruit salad plate
	Melba toast—2 slices
	Margarine—1 pat
	Tea or coffee
Dinner	Broiled chicken breast à l'orange
	Fresh peas with baby onions
	Chicory, endive, and cucumber salad with low-calorie French dressing
	Pineapple chunks (no sugar)
	Bread—1 slice and 1 pat margarine
	Tea or coffee
Between meals	Low calorie beverages
	Celery and carrot strips
	Fresh fruit—one serving
Bed-time	Nonfat milk—one glass
	Crackers—2
	Cheese—1 ounce

If a cocktail before dinner is in order or a highball will be consumed during the evening, omit the cheese and half of the margarine.

Another lady writes that she has been told to lose weight because of impending surgery on her hip. She has lost all but six pounds of the prescribed reduction, but seems to be stuck at this level and needs some suggestions. Although she said that she has been eating a 1,000-calorie diet and exercising, she has been unable to reach her goal of 140 pounds. Certainly it does seem that the last five pounds are always the most difficult to lose. Even so, it should be possible to lose as much as two pounds per week if one sticks tenaciously to 1,000 calories daily. The chances are that the 1,000 calories are just too limiting for many dieters to be able to follow for very long. Therefore, a diet supplying between 1,200 and 1,300 calories daily is a bit more flexible and satisfying, while still allowing a weight loss of roughly a pound per week for most people. Listed below is such a diet:

Breakfast	4 ounces orange juice or ½-grapefruit
	Cereal with skim milk

Lunch	1 small cup vegetable soup
	Open-faced sandwich (2 slices lean roast beef and 1 slice bread with 1 teaspoon margarine or mayonnaise)
	½-cup shredded cabbage and green pepper with vinegar dressing
	Tea or coffee (no sugar or cream)
Afternoon snack	1 glass skim milk
	1 medium apple
Dinner	4 ounces broiled fish with lemon
	1 small baked potato with 1 teaspoon margarine
	1 serving broccoli
	Sliced tomato and lettuce salad with low-calorie dressing
	Sugar-free gelatin dessert with ½-sliced banana
	Tea or coffee (no cream or sugar)
Bed-time	1 glass skim milk or beer
	2 crackers or pretzels

AND NOW FOR THE MEN

Here is a suggested plan for men who need to lose weight gradually and yet maintain a reasonable level of activity. Specifically, this day's menu plan was developed for a 54-year-old man in good health, but whose weight of 180 pounds needs to be reduced by approximately 30 pounds. A 2,000-calorie diet is recommended as allowing an encouraging weight loss while providing a reasonable degree of satisfaction and retraining of the appetite.

Breakfast	Citrus fruit, juice, or tomato juice
	Cereal with skim milk and banana
	Toast or roll with jam
Mid-morning	Coffee or soft drink
Lunch	Soup and crackers
	Sandwich
	Fruit
	Beverage
Mid-afternoon	Coffee, tea, soft drink, or skim milk
Dinner	Plain meat, such as pot roast (4 ounces)
	Baked potato—1 medium
	Cooked vegetable
	Salad of raw vegetables
	Dish of ice cream
	Beverage
Before bed	Beer and pretzels or skim milk and crackers

With the preceding diets for taking off some weight, it is important that the dieter also be physically active—taking brisk walks, jogging easily, or using the muscles in some type of good workout. This results in better muscle tone and increased utilization of energy. By taking the stairs when going up two or three flights, playing tennis, swimming, or playing racquetball, or other favored activity, you can also increase your energy expenditure. Moderate and regular exercise is important in weight reduction and it does burn up calories.

THE FATS IN YOUR LIFE

Butter and margarine are discussed almost as if they were poison by many dieters, so a few remarks about these products may help in deciding what types of fats to buy. Any product that is labeled "margarine" must contain a minimum of 80 percent fat, a value consistent with that occurring naturally in butter. The identification of a margarine as containing less saturated fat or being higher in unsaturated fat does not change the amount of fat that is required in the standard margarines by law. Thus, butter and margarine contribute nine calories per gram of pure fat, just as the various vegetable oils and other fats in the diet do. However, there are products on the market which are identified as "diet margarines." These generally contain about half the amount of fat that regular margarines provide, i.e., about 45 percent rather than 80 percent, and thus contribute only about half the calories. This is accomplished by adding water to the formulation, which makes these diet margarines poorly suited to a number of food preparations.

Pure fat contains over twice as many calories per gram as either carbohydrates or proteins (nine calories per gram compared with approximately four calories per gram of either carbohydrate or protein). Of course, diet margarines and also whipped butter or whipped margarine will contribute fewer calories per tablespoon than the regular products because of the volume represented by water and/or air, neither of which contributes energy. Whipped butter and whipped margarine, as well as some types of ice cream, are simply puffed up by whipping air into them. Thus, when a serving based on volume is eaten, one actually gets far fewer calories than with the unwhipped product. Obviously, this is another way of cutting back on the calories from fats in your diet.

Yet another fat-containing market item with an eye to the dieter's problem is a Neufchatel cheese, a creamy type of cheese which is 30 percent lower in fat and 30 percent higher in protein, yet contains 25 percent fewer calories than cream cheese. With this Neufchatel cheese product, you can put the same amount on a cracker as cream cheese, and yet end up with 25 percent fewer calories.

While most of us probably don't eat enough cream cheese for this single item to lessen our energy intake much, when the same activity takes place with a dozen other foods, these little savings in calories will add up to a significant figure for the dieter. A new word has come into foods and beverages—"light". We now have light beers, light wines, light spreads, light canned fruits, etc. These refer to foods with fewer calories due to less alcohol, less fat, and less sugar content.

Be on the lookout for "light foods" lower in energy, particularly those with less fat, because the greatest savings can be made by reducing the fat in foods.

NONFAT AND LOW-FAT MILK—A SIGNIFICANT DIET AID

At one time nonfat or skim milk was considered to be practically unfit for humans, and it was usual in some dairy regions to find that cream was removed from milk and sold to creameries, while the remaining skim milk was used as food for the livestock. This happened back in the days when nobody had heard of cholesterol, and hard physical exercise was an accepted part of living. Today, for all too many people, the hardest exercise all day is walking out to the kitchen quickly to get a snack during television commercials. As you are well aware, this sedentary life that most of us lead has helped to produce a good many overweight Americans. Now naturally we would all like to look like those deliciously thin models in magazines, but it is just too hard to give up some of those high-calorie goodies we love so much. No matter how much weight you are hoping to lose, it is desirable to have some milk or milk products each day to be well nourished. If you drink two glasses of whole milk daily, those two glasses of milk will contribute about 320 calories all by themselves. If you were trying to go on a 1,000-calorie diet, these two glasses of milk alone would contribute almost a third of the entire day's diet. Now, if instead you drink two glasses of skim or nonfat milk, those glasses contain only 180 calories together, or less than a fifth of the energy in a 1,000-calorie diet. This probably sounds so good that you may immediately be suspicious and wonder what the catch is. Just what are you giving up when you substitute skim milk for whole milk in your diet? The answer basically is "fat"—milk fat and your fat. This sounds really good, doesn't it; but what happens to the nutrients when milk is skimmed? If you were to examine a table showing the amounts of the various nutrients in skim milk and whole milk, you would find that the protein, minerals, B vitamins, and carbohydrate levels are just about the same in skim and whole milk. Vitamin A, a fat-soluble vitamin, is present only in whole milk unless the skim milk has been "fortified" with this vitamin, which it should be. The same general comments apply to the other major fat-soluble vitamin—vitamin D. The label will tell the story concerning the addition of these vitamins.

In short then, skim milk or low fat milk fortified with vitamins A and D are very suitable foods in your diet and can well be used in place of whole milk if you are seeking to limit your weight or lose weight.

Of course, the flavor of skim milk is not as rich as whole milk because the fat has been removed. Something of a compromise in this regard is provided by low fat milks, which have between ⅓ and ⅔ of their fat removed to yield low fat milks with a fat content of 1 to 2 percent, rather than the 3 to 3½ percent of whole milk. But don't be overwhelmed by the promotion of 1 percent fat milks as being 99 percent fat-free. They are, but then whole milk is 97 percent fat-free! A more reasonable way to promote 1 percent fat milks would be to say that 66 percent of the fat has been removed. But Madison Avenue prefers the looks of 99 percent fat-free.

By cutting out calories in such ways as this, you can begin to control your weight sensibly. Compare this approach with the reports of two ladies who tried using pills.

WILL POWER VS. PILL POWER

A 27-year-old mother of two young children writes that she has been taking amphetamine tablets to reduce her appetite for almost two years. She said, "I tried to stop taking them, and in one week I gained about ten pounds. I just couldn't seem to stop eating all the time. I have no will power. Do you think it is all in my mind? Will these have an effect on my heart? I am about 30 pounds overweight. Will the continuation of these pills be harmful?" A second lady reported that she reduced her weight from 180 pounds to 128 by going to a doctor who gave her pills, shots, and a diet. When she reached 128 pounds, she stopped both her visits to the doctor and the diet he had given her. She promptly regained her former obese figure and wondered why this happened.

One certainly must question the wisdom of taking amphetamines or other drugs for weight reduction on a daily basis for long periods of time, although some people may find them helpful in reducing the appetite during the first month or so to help get them started on a good program of weight reduction. However, they should only be used on the advice and under the supervision of a physician.

Eventually, it is necessary to change one's pattern of living by eating less and getting more exercise if weight loss is to be accomplished and maintained permanently.

THE "FAST" APPROACH

In spite of all that has been written about sensible diets for losing weight, many people still are convinced that the best way for them to lose weight is to eat nothing at all. Since the goal of any diet should be learning to live *with* food, not without it, we can hardly recommend fasting as a means of establishing permanent weight control. At best, a fasting diet (with or without protein supplements) can only be considered a temporary crutch; at worst, it can be downright dangerous. Approximately 80 deaths, probably related to fasting with hydrolyzed protein supplements, have been investigated by the Food and Drug Administration.

No type of fasting diet should be undertaken without the aid of a physician. It would be best to do this only in a hospital. Metabolic changes are numerous and not always predictable. Fasting for more than two days can cause slowing of the heart rate and a decrease in muscle strength and coordination, so that physical performance declines significantly with every 10 to 15 percent loss of body weight, advises D. R. Young, an M.D. and research scientist with the National Aeronautics and Space Administration. Although people have survived losses of 50 to 60 percent of initial body weight during chronic semi-starvation, according to Dr. Young, this is "probably within the range of the lethal limit." Interestingly, only 30 percent of the fat lost is from tissues under the skin, while 50 percent is from tissues supporting various body organs and the intestines, which creates a very dangerous situation.

With little or no carbohydrate, the body enters a state of ketosis, whereby alcohol-like chemicals called ketones build up in the blood and urine. Also, the protein lost is from the heart, liver, kidneys, and skin, as well as from muscles of the arms and legs. These are other dangerous situations.

Increasingly, total fasting is being replaced by "modified fasting" diets, which include a protein supplement (not hydrolyzed), along with additional vitamins and minerals. The addition of protein partially prevents the body from raiding the protein in its own muscles and vital organs, and forces it to use only its stores of fat. However, many of the protein supplements are less than useless, because they are of poor quality and in fact are not superior to powdered milk mixed with water. Powdered milk contains a "complete" protein and certainly is easier on your pocketbook than any of the supplementary protein products on the market.

However, fasting diets are likely to be accompanied by unpleasant side effects such as hair loss, muscle weakness, dizziness, nausea, headaches, gallbladder flareups, bad breath, difficulty in keeping warm, menstrual irregularity, constipation, and even nervous disorders, if they are used for as little as two days. This is true regardless of the source of the protein.

Fasting is sometimes claimed to rid the blood of various substances. Unfortunately, the substances can include vitamins and necessary minerals, which are lost with the breakdown and death of cells. Since no nutrients are being consumed in fasting, these lost nutrients are not replenished.

People with malfunctions of the liver, kidneys, or heart—malfunctions which may not be known to the individual—risk great potential danger from fasting because of the extensive changes that take place in the body and its chemistry. Even ulcerative colitis has been observed in fasting patients.

Fasting diets can modify the effects of medications for such chronic conditions as diabetes and high blood pressure. This is yet another reason for needing medical supervision if you are tempted to fast.

Few physicians will recommend any type of fast unless the patient is 50 or more pounds overweight. In that case, the goal will be to experience an initial speedy weight loss (mostly water) in order to provide an impetus for continuing a sensible long-term weight loss program.

If you feel that a starvation-type regimen is the only solution for you, your physician will perform a physical examination as well as blood and other laboratory tests to determine whether you can undertake such a diet with relative safety—and RELATIVE safety is the best guarantee a doctor can provide.

Weekly check-ups will be necessary throughout the fast; follow-up maintenance visits also will be required if the weight loss is to continue successfully.

It must be pointed out, however, that studies conducted at the University of California over a 9-year period have shown that less than 6 percent of the dieters who underwent total fasting had maintained reduced weights at the end of nine years. The poorest records in the studies were among persons who had been obese since early childhood, which gives added impetus to parents to help their children develop well-balanced, well-proportioned dietary patterns. We do not recommend the use of starvation or "modified" fasting diets because they are too dangerous for most people to follow by themselves.

Most important for any dieter is to learn to live with food, not without it, and to consume a balanced diet from the Basic Four Food Groups (fruits and vegetables, milk and cheese, cereals and breads, meats-poultry-fish). In short, the dieter needs to learn to adhere to a maintenance diet based on a wide range of food. This diet will enable people to achieve and maintain ideal weight and to have the best possible health. Portion size, particularly of meat and the milk group, should be adjusted to reach the weight reduction and maintenance goals.

FADS AND OTHER DANGEROUS DIETS

Many people, in their efforts to lose weight, stray far from the safe and sure methods and fall for various diet fads, which are neither effective nor safe as a solution to weight control. Some go so far as to consider extreme and dangerous methods for losing weight. Some of these methods which should be avoided are discussed below.

Human chorionic gonadotropin (HCG) is a growth hormone extracted from the urine of pregnant women. The HCG diet calls for 500 calories per day plus daily visits to the local HCG clinic for a hormone shot and a pep talk.

Dr. Albert T. Simeons used HCG in the treatment of young boys suffering from Fröhlich's syndrome—a condition which caused boys to accumulate feminizing fat on the hips, buttocks, and thighs, making them look like girls. Injections of HCG helped reduce this fat. Dr. Simeons and his colleagues reasoned that, with the liberated fat as a major source of nourishment, would-be dieters could also benefit from the drug. And thus began a chain of Simeons Weight Reduction Institutes, followed by the Kennedy Diet Centers and other individual "diet clinics" around the country based on the HCG technique. Numerous lawsuits have emerged as the realization grew that many of these clinics were operated by non-professional individuals who paid certain doctors to refer patients to the HCG program.

The diet itself does indeed cause weight loss, but there is no evidence that HCG has anything to do with it. The diet includes only 500 calories per day. Therefore, the same side effects and inherent dangers are present in the use of this diet as in any other diet too low in energy. Also, these problems are often compounded by inadequate medical supervision.

Furthermore, HCG causes its own side effects—headache, restlessness, and depression, among others. Studies by the Food and Drug Administration concluded that "there are no scientifically adequate, well-controlled clinical studies appearing in medical literature which establish the safety and efficiency of HCG in the treatment of obesity." Deliberate and unnecessary exposure to the unknown, possibly long-term effects of such a potent hormone is just not smart.

Surgical diets represent another approach to weight control which is loaded with potential difficulties. For example, a 322-pound English male nurse, whose normal daily diet included a whole chicken, four sandwiches, a pound of beef, dozens of slices of toast, a pound of chocolate, gallons of sweet coffee and tea and whatever else struck his fancy, reportedly had his mouth wired shut by a dental surgeon. For 112 days he sipped milk and lost 105 pounds.

And so began a new weight-reducing technique—surgically locking the jaw. Sometimes the diet included only milk. Other times all the components of a normal meal were liquified in a blender and sipped through a straw. Just because food was in a liquid form did not mean that the energy intake was always limited.

This is a hazardous procedure because, in addition to the obvious handicaps of not being able to open the mouth, there is the possibility of sputum or vomitus being inhaled into the lungs, as well as the probability of tooth decay, shifting of tooth position, and gum disease.

Even more drastic than this procedure is an operation known as *jejuno-ileal bypass*. With this technique, a portion of the intestines is clamped off (or occasionally removed), thus preventing proper digestion of food and reducing absorption of nutrients and energy. This is the only diet which allows you to eat as much as you wish and still lose weight, but the dangers are great. It is a difficult, high-risk operation used only on patients who are so obese that their lives are already in jeopardy. About five percent do not even survive the operation itself.

The renewed interest in acupuncture has fostered a surgical gimmick called *staplepuncture*. The theory here is that there are appetite-suppressing nerves running from the stomach to the ears. With the surgical implantation of special metal clips into the ears, the dieter supposedly has only to wiggle the clips when he feels hungry, and his stomach will think it has been fed. Food intake is limited to 400 calories daily, which of course causes weight loss.

A more recent surgical procedure is that of actually making the stomach smaller by a third to a half by stapling off a portion of it. Thus one becomes "full" with less food because there is less space to fill. And if one overeats, some of the food will be rejected by vomiting. One soon learns to eat less! Currently, stapling off a portion of the stomach is the best and safest surgical procedure for dealing with extreme obesity.

Surgical methods of weight control, as you can see, are extreme, sometimes dangerous, and not to be considered for use by the average dieter. It is much easier to use mind control than surgical control of weight and to modify eating habits by consuming fewer calories and burning up more of them.

REDUCING DIET POTPOURRI

Readers ask innumerable questions about the current dieting fads. One writer asked, "Are the Drinking Man's Diet, the Low Carbohydrate Diet, and the Diet for Fat Pilots all the same, and was the latter devised and used at the USAF Academy?" The answer, briefly, is that they are all essentially the same, and the Air Force Academy had nothing to do with any of the diets. We have not been able to trace the rumor to its source which linked the Air Force Academy with that diet.

Since various versions of the Low Carbohydrate Diet keep cropping up, it seems appropriate to include a reader's query and the answer to it in this book. The reader inquired, "What is the Drinking Man's Diet, and what do you think of it?" The answer is—not much. The Drinking Man's Diet is nothing but a marinated version of the Calories Don't Count Diet, but with even more nutritional nonsense, if that is possible (and it seems to be). The more nonsensical part of this diet is the implication that because most alcoholic beverages (whiskey and gin, for example) do not contain carbohydrate, they can be consumed generously without putting on weight. This rationale appears to ignore the known fact that pure alcohol contributes almost twice as much energy, gram per gram, as is contributed by carbohydrates. In fact, alcohol provides seven calories per gram while carbohydrate contributes four calories per gram.

The whimsy of this diet can be seen when it is recognized that the diet restricts carbohydrate to an intake of only 60 grams daily (compared to the usual intake of 300 to 400 grams daily). This great reduction in carbohydrate intake results in a relative increase in the proportion of the energy derived from protein and fat. Such a circumstance will lead to ketosis, a potentially dangerous condition, if the diet is pursued diligently.

In addition to the potential health hazards of such a diet, nutritionists are critical of fad diets because they are so narrow that much of the pleasure of eating is eliminated from life. When this is true, few people will persist long enough to effect the desired weight change, and their regular eating pattern which caused the obesity will be resumed. For success in dieting and weight control, permanent changes in dietary habits, yet changes which afford pleasure without weight gain, need to be made.

CALORIES DO COUNT!

With the emphasis on high protein diets, low carbohydrate reducing diet plans, and on and·on ad infinitum, a few words on the sources of calories in the diet may help in sorting out some of the confusion and contradictions you hear.

Let's start with a typical adult diet of 3,000 calories for a male. The energy will be available approximately as follows: 40 percent from fats, 45 percent from carbohydrates, and 15 percent from proteins. Obviously, these percentages may vary from day to day and from person to person, but usually they will be close to these values.

Thus, simple arithmetic shows that a typical diet of 3,000 calories will provide approximately 1,200 calories from fat, 1,350 from carbohydrates, and 450 from proteins. Now, to get these amounts of energy into grams of fat, carbohydrate, and protein, the fat calories have to be divided by 9 and the carbohydrate and protein by 4. Thus, a 3,000-calorie diet will contain about 133 grams of fat, 338 grams of carbohydrate, and 112 grams of protein. If you prefer to think of weights in ounces, simply divide by 30 to get a rough approximation.

The same arithmetic can be applied to a 1,500-calorie reducing diet, which would result in a weight loss of approximately a pound and a half a week for most males. In this situation, the diet would contain about 66 grams of fat, 169 grams of carbohydrate, and 56 grams of protein.

Sixty grams of carbohydrate are specified frequently as the amount allowed in a low carbohydrate reducing diet. Note how this small quantity compares with the 169 grams included in the 1,500-calorie reducing diet just mentioned. The limitations become even more apparent when we look at this amount of carbohydrate in terms of actual food. For instance, a quart of milk provides approximately 48 grams of carbohydrate, and two servings of hash provide about 12 grams. Although these two items total 60 grams of carbohydrate, they are a long way from being a good diet. Here's another example: A half cup of lima beans provides 21 grams of carbohydrate, one ear of corn adds 20, and a small potato 19 grams, for a total of 60 grams of carbohydrate, but a nutritionally incomplete diet.

On such a severely restricted diet, most fruits, vegetables, and cereals are excluded or greatly restricted. This is most unfortunate because they are important sources of many vitamins and minerals. Cereals and legumes also are comparatively inexpensive sources of protein.

A workable diet should include specific suggestions for breakfast, lunch, dinner, and snacks and should provide variety throughout the week. Any diet that uses a narrow range of foods almost exclusively will be very monotonous. In addition, it has the disadvantage of not retraining your habits into a pattern that can be enjoyed for a lifetime of proper weight control. Low carbohydrate diets are but one of the wrinkles that need to be ironed out in the realm of diets to lose weight.

A FAD DIET POTLUCK

Through the years, many types of diets have soared to the forefront of cocktail party conversation, retreated to general oblivion, and then advanced again, generally in a readily recognizable form.

Is it true that grapefruit serves as a catalyst in burning fats (as the Mayo Diet states) so that a person can "stuff" himself

with any foods except starches and sugars and still lose weight?

No, that is not true, and the so-called "Mayo Diet" has never had any connection with the well known Mayo Clinic in Rochester, Minnesota. It is strictly an odd diet. Grapefruit is a fine food and a rich source of vitamin C, but it does not have any unique properties for burning fats. It is not a big yellow spark plug igniting fats!

I read that the grapefruit diet is dangerous to one's health. I am sending you a copy for your evaluation of it and its safety. If this isn't safe, what is a safe diet?

Most "way out" diets like the grapefruit diet are not dangerous because few people will stick to them for more than a few days. The concern about this diet is not because of the emphasis on grapefruit, but because of the large intake of eggs and fat. Eggs are an excellent food from the standpoint of nutritive value, but the yolk is a rich source of cholesterol, and in some individuals the intake of cholesterol should be restricted. Most of the so-called scientific comments that usually accompany the grapefruit diet, including those you mentioned in your letter, are pretty much nonsense. It would be interesting to know how the fad of the grapefruit diet ever got started.

Do you claim that it is not true that by eating fat you burn fat? Also, are products made from safflower oil nutritionally superior to those made from corn oil? And are these oils an aid in maintaining weight? Since safflower oil products are more expensive than some of the other margarines and salad oils, I wonder if I am wasting my hard-earned money.

Eating fat does not help one burn or metabolize fat. Safflower oil does contain more linoleic acid, the principal polyunsaturated fatty acid, than some of the common vegetable oils, such as corn, cottonseed, and soya, but there is no evidence that it makes any difference in one's weight or general health as to which oil is used in typical diets in this country. In general, the choice of safflower, corn, cottonseed, or soya oils is largely one of palatability to the consumer and cost.

Some of the new diets recommend protein powder mixed with milk or fruit juice for breakfast and lunch, and then a well-balanced meal for dinner. You are also supposed to add B vitamins and unsaturated oil. What do you think of this plan?

Dietary fads such as this were popular several years ago. They keep coming and going. The protein powders are unnecessary, a great waste of money and, in fact, are a real nutritional rip-off. Most of us eat twice as much protein as we need, anyway. There is protein in that glass of milk that you mentioned for breakfast, and there is protein in the meat in your well balanced dinner.

Having one good meal at dinnertime and only a glass of milk, juice, maybe an instant breakfast food, or a snack for the other two meals may be perfectly satisfactory. There is no reason to waste your money on protein powders, extra vitamins, and unsaturated oils. Some foods from each of the Basic Four Food Groups should be included in your daily plan so that you will get the variety of nutrients you need. A regular potency, one-a-day type vitamin supplement is probably not necessary but can be used if you are eating a diet well below 2,000 calories daily.

My friend tells me she feels terrific since she has been using a high-potency milkshake for breakfast, but she tells me it contains 40,000 I.U. of vitamin A and 3,000 of vitamin D. Isn't it dangerous to take so much vitamin A and vitamin D?

It certainly is dangerous. Those levels are each about ten times more than is needed, and if continued for several months, your friend may experience health problems. In a child, the time for creating these problems would be shorter.

Milkshakes are perfectly good food and can be a part of any good diet, but there is no reason to fortify them with added nutrients. It would be a good idea for your friend to eat a more typical breakfast in order to give her teeth, gums, and jaws a little exercise.

Are all the liquid proteins harmful? I've heard that some have caused death.

Deaths have been caused by use of the liquid protein made from hydrolyzed collagen. This substance is one of the poorest proteins, from a nutritional standpoint, and should never be used as the only source of nutrition. There are other liquid proteins made from milk and soya protein, which are sound nutritionally.

However, in our opinion, liquid proteins are seldom necessary or even desirable unless, for some reason, a person is unable to eat food normally. Therefore, we consider them to be a waste of money for the dieter and when used in a modified fasting regimen with a total daily caloric intake of only 400 to 500 calories daily to be very dangerous.

A liquid protein diet, popular on the West Coast, is known as the Cambridge Diet. It is sold from door to door by sales personnel known as Cambridge Counselors. We think it dangerous and should be avoided "like the plague," and would bet our last nickel that few Cambridge Counselors are professionally qualified in health or nutrition.

There is no liquid protein diet that has been proven to be successful over the long term for either losing weight or for one's health. In fact, liquid protein diets have proven to be dangerous and are reported to have been associated with at least 80 deaths. The best diet for losing weight (and also the least expensive) is the "less diet"—eat less, spend less, weigh less!

If you really want to lose weight, try eating half-portions at each meal, taking small bites and chewing longer. Try to retain the normal balance of carbohydrates, proteins, and fat which is recommended for good health. This may mean reducing your intake of fat somewhat in comparison to the reduction in carbohydrate and protein. Remember the maxim, "Eat slowly and lose slowly"; a healthy diet plan for the long pull is a gradual one which retrains dietary habits without going to extremes.

Trying to keep excess pounds off is a constant battle for me. Lunches eaten at work are my greatest downfall. How can a working woman eat a diet lunch?

You are not alone with this problem. Readers tell us that lunchtime is devastating for many dieters. However, it need not be this way. To cope calorically with a working lunch, you have to be creative, exercise a significant amount of will power (or perhaps, more accurately, "won't power"), and follow some suggestions.

To begin, let us warn you against skipping lunch. To meet the demands of any challenging job, you must maintain your mental and physical energy at a high level. Because the hours between breakfast and dinner are long and busy, your body requires some refueling midway. The trick is to make sure that the fuel you take in is not a caloric disaster.

Do you brown-bag your lunch? Sandwiches can be part of your diet routine, but use only one piece of bread, avoid the use of butter or other spreads, and steer clear of delicatessen meats high in calories and fat. Poultry, diet cheeses, tuna, and egg salad (with just a smidgen of mayonnaise, but lots of celery and spices) are attractive, tasty alternatives. Flesh out the sandwich with lettuce, sprouts, and tomato slices to add color, texture, and bulk. One of us (FJS) routinely eats only a half-sandwich for lunch, the other half goes to his secretary!

If your office boasts a refrigerator, the low-calorie luncheon possibilities are virtually endless. Salads, yogurt, and cottage cheese are some favorite lunchtime carry-alongs.

Delicatessen lunches are the diet downfall of many people. However, you can still have a delicatessen lunch that will not be a diet disaster. Most delis sell salads which feature lettuce or spinach. Some even have fresh fruit salads. If eaten with only a small amount of dressing, they can form the basis of a tasty, low-calorie luncheon. Supplemented by melba toast or a few saltines and finished off with fresh fruit or low fat yogurt, the delicatessen lunch is tasty and full of variety.

Eating in restaurants is particularly difficult for many dieters because temptations are present at every course. First, the generous amount of butter available for rolls needs to be avoided. Then high-fat main dishes need to be avoided, and finally, the calorie-rich desserts must be resisted.

Lists of appetizers usually include melon or shrimp cocktail, two tasty and filling selections that are relatively low in calories. Water-based soups are also good choices. Eating an appetizer makes it easier to eat less during the rest of the meal.

A broiled poultry or fish item is the best selection for a main course. Ask the waitress to have it done without added fat. Avoid French fries. Instead, ask for a small baked or boiled potato or two other vegetables.

Cakes and pies are definite "no-no" foods for dieters, but you can still treat yourself to something while others are indulging. Try an interesting new tea or perhaps some fresh strawberries to end your meal. And remember to consult the appetizer list. That fresh fruit cup can be eaten at the end of the meal as well as at the beginning!

Losing weight has always been difficult for me, and I find that the special diet foods make it a little easier. However, with food prices rising, I now find it very difficult to squeeze higher-priced items into my food budget. Do you have any answers?

Diet foods ARE more expensive. In fact, some estimates say they are about 23 percent higher than their non-diet supermarket counterparts. The way out is to turn supermarket shelf foods into diet foods.

Buy water-packed tuna from the canned fish section rather than the dietetic water-packed from the diet section. Use fresh vegetables in season, then switch to frozen or canned. Unless you are on a medical low-salt diet, you do not need the special ones labeled "dietetic". The trick is to select only lower calorie vegetables, steering clear of starchy beans and corn.

Fresh fruits are less expensive during some parts of the year and usually are tastier than the dietetic canned fruits. Check your prices and compare to see which is the better value for you. Some of the popular, name brand canned fruits and juices are now being packed without added sugar. Reading your labels carefully is the key to saving here.

Make up your own frozen diet dinners. By cooking in quantity at one time and then freezing in individual servings for later, you'll get some of the convenience and the portion size control you seek, but at a lower price.

Instead of frying in butter or oil, try the no-stick spray designed to be used on certain frying pans that are becoming increasingly popular. One such can will go a long way, while also saving you the cost of the oil and the calories the oil would provide.

I'm desperately trying to lose weight. How many calories do I have to give up in order to lose one pound?

A pound of body fat represents the equivalent of about 3,500 calories. Thus, a daily deficit of 500 calories will lead to an average weekly loss of one pound.

Do you feel that there is anything unhealthy about going on a 500 to 800-calorie-a-day diet?

For relatively active people, a daily intake of less than 1,500 calories for men and 1,000 for women is poorly tolerated. Keep in mind that you can lose weight effectively by both reducing calorie intake and increasing caloric expenditure, that is, by exercising. For instance, if you decrease calorie intake from food and drink by 300 per day and increase caloric expenditure by 200 calories per day, you will accomplish the same effect as a decrease of 500 calories in the diet. This approach is generally more acceptable and easier to follow than severe calorie restriction alone.

Are diuretics useful in dieting?

No, and they may be harmful to your health. Salt restriction may be a more sound measure than the use of diuretics to prevent excessive water retention. This is particularly true for middleaged and older women and sedentary persons who often have a marked tendency to retain fluids.

What about "formula diets"?

These became popular in the past couple of decades and offer the advantage of providing a simple, rigid regimen that does not need to be based on any knowledge of food and food values. They may be useful at the beginning of a weight control program or for a one-meal-a-day replacement in some instances. However, they have the definite disadvantage of being a very boring way of feeding yourself. Formula diets, therefore, do not provide a continuing solution to weight problems.

How many calories do we generally burn each hour?

That depends on what you are doing during that hour and how big you are. If you are sitting, you will burn about 90 calories; standing, about 120; walking, 220; golfing, 300; playing tennis, bowling, or rowing, 500. Remember that weight seldom is reduced by exercise alone. You have to be wise about what you eat as well as what you do. You cannot pay calorically for a long, cold gin and tonic by a few swings of the golf club.

THE CALORIES IN YOUR LIFE

A lady who described herself as an average homemaker with two small children asked how many calories she should be eating each day. According to her description, she does her own housework, cares for the children, and mows the lawn or takes an occasional walk for exercise. Other than that, she felt she got virtually no exercise because exercising with television was inconvenient and boring. She concluded by requesting calorie information for the inactive housewife like herself.

To anyone trying to keep up with this average "inactive" housewife, this lady might have some difficulty convincing the observer that she really was inactive. Caring for two small children and doing housework can require a lot of energy. The National Research Council recommends 2,000 calories per day for women who regularly have average activity. Actually, the number of calories needed daily is influenced by many things, such as sex, age, and amount of activity. The following chart, excerpted from the Food and Nutrition Board, National Academy of Sciences-National Research Council's 1980 revision of the Recommended Dietary Allowances, gives a rough guide to the number of calories needed by individuals of various ages. People who sit a lot or lead generally inactive lives need an amount closer to the lower end of the recommended range, and those people who exercise considerably on their job or heatedly pursue active hobbies require more calories to maintain weight.

MEAN HEIGHTS AND WEIGHTS AND RECOMMENDED ENERGY INTAKE[1]

Category	Age	Weight		Height		Energy needs (with range) cal
		kg	lb	cm	in	
Infants	0.0–0.5	6	13	60	24	kg × 115 (95–145)
	0.5–1.0	9	20	71	28	kg × 105 (80–135)
Children	1–3	13	29	90	35	1300 (900–1800)
	4–6	20	44	112	44	1700 (1300–2300)
	7–10	28	62	132	52	2400 (1650–3300)
Males	11–14	45	99	157	62	2700 (2000–3700)
	15–18	66	145	176	69	2800 (2100–3900)
	19–22	70	154	177	70	2900 (2500–3300)
	23–50	70	154	178	70	2700 (2300–3100)
	51–75	70	154	178	70	2400 (2000–2800)
	76+	70	154	178	70	2050 (1650–2450)
Females	11–14	46	101	157	62	2200 (1500–3000)
	15–18	55	120	163	64	2100 (1200–3000)
	19–22	55	120	163	64	2100 (1700–2500)
	23–50	55	120	163	64	2000 (1600–2400)
	51–75	55	120	163	64	1800 (1400–2200)
	76+	55	120	163	64	1600 (1200–2000)
Pregnancy						+300
Lactation						+500

[1] From *Recommended Dietary Allowances*. Food and Nutrition Board, National Academy of Sciences-National Research Council. Washington, D.C., 9th Ed., 1980.

One of the questions about dieting is whether or not it is all right to drink water. Many people think that drinking water will cause them to remain fat even though they are eating a diet considerably lower in calories than they normally do. Water does not make one fat, but it may make you heavier than you actually are if the water is retained at higher than normal levels in the tissues and not eliminated efficiently by the kidneys. After all, water is "a pint a pound the world around." One of the reasons for a low salt diet is to minimize the amount of water retained in the body tissues. And don't accept the idea that drinking ice water will help you lose weight because of the calories used up in bringing the water to body temperature. The number of calories required for this is pretty small. We can't advise just how many calories you need daily because of the influence of activity, age, sex, and height, but you can use the previous table plus noting your tendency to maintain, gain, or lose weight to estimate your requirement.

WATCH OUT FOR THAT COCKTAIL!

With so much comment on dieting and selection for weight loss, a word of caution about cocktails clearly is in order. Unlike water, that "see-through" cocktail is just another enticing way of getting more calories into your body. In fact, it can be a rather concentrated source of energy.

You can make an estimate of the calories in various cocktails if you are armed with a bit of information. Remember that alcohol contributes about 210 calories per ounce or 7 calories per gram. Since the alcoholic content of your cocktail is not 100 percent, more sophisticated calculations are necessary to arrive at a more precise figure. The alcoholic content of most hard liquors (whiskey, gin, vodka, etc.) is reported in what is termed "proof". You can convert the proof of alcohol to a percentage value by dividing the proof figure by two. Multiply this percentage times the ounces of alcohol times 210 to find the calories contributed by the alcohol in a cocktail. Simple enough, but often with a discouraging answer. Also, don't forget that some drinks have sugar added, and it is difficult to ignore the calorie-laden temptations, such as fried egg rolls, nuts, sour cream dips and chips, and other cocktail hour fare. Now, if you really are interested in the calories in your cocktail, but don't wish to do that arithmetic yourself, a good figure to keep in mind is that an average cocktail or highball provides between 115 and 230 calories, depending on whether it contains one or two ounces of the alcoholic ingredient.

CARBOHYDRATES—FRIEND OR FOE?

Many people think carbohydrates are the cause of their weight problem and promptly assume that starches and sugars must be eliminated from their diets when they are trying to reduce. Several of the fad diets further reinforce this notion by severely restricting carbohydrates in the diet. The weight loss this engenders is mainly water loss and provides a potentially dangerous and temporary solution to the problem of obesity.

Ketosis develops when the body receives so little carbohydrate that metabolism cannot proceed normally. Without carbohydrate in low-calorie diets, fat deposits in the tissues are broken down to provide necessary energy. This breakdown happens at a faster rate than can be handled in the body, and substances known as ketone bodies build up in the body. These ketones interfere with the body's normal acid/base balance and must be excreted in the urine. The result is a substantial loss of water (and therefore, weight). To prevent severe dehydration and to assure sufficient fluid for removal of the ketone bodies, water intake must be maintained at an unusually high level.

Ketosis is an abnormal body state. The real and inherent danger of toying with body chemistry lies in the possible precipitation of a pre-existing medical condition. Many cases are on record of chemical manipulation having led directly to disorders of the heart, liver, kidneys, and gastrointestinal tract.

Although it is true that most Americans consume far too much fat, some fat is necessary to promote a satisfied feeling after a meal. Some carbohydrate in the diet is necessary to metabolize the fat properly and avoid ketosis. Therefore, we say that moderation and a healthful, nutritionally balanced diet which is varied and enjoyable and sprinkled liberally with common sense are the ingredients of a successful weight reduction program.

While we are thinking about weight control and a varied diet, let's look at a few other questions people have asked about calories in foods.

Please tell me if papaya and mango are to be avoided on a reducing diet. Are these more fattening than cantaloupe or watermelon? How large a piece provides 100 calories?

No foods need be avoided on a reducing diet. Fresh fruits are frequently favored in reducing diets because they contain lots of water, little fat, and hence are rather low in energy. Mangoes have about 50 percent more calories than papayas because they contain more fat and sugar. Mangoes are about the same as nectarines in caloric value, and papayas are comparable to melons. Five ounces of a mango would provide about 100 calories, and it would take seven ounces of papaya for the same number of calories. These are generous servings. For comparison, three ounces of chicken or turkey (a small serving) would approximate 250 calories, and three ounces (also a small serving) of beef provides about 400 calories.

A Midwestern homemaker writes, "Please could you tell me which foods are high in nutrition, but low in calories so that I could prepare long-lasting meals for my husband? At present he seems to need a snack, but he also needs to lose weight." Her solution is to serve meats, fish, eggs, milk and its products, peas, beans, and cereals, but in modest portions. The snack could continue, but it should be an item saved from the dinner meal rather than being an extra food.

Although I know that I need to restrict food intake, I still nibble. Would it help me to avoid nibbling if I developed a hobby to keep me busy?

Actually, nibbling can be an acceptable part of a diet plan. A controlled nibble about half an hour before a meal dulls the appetite and helps to make you less hungry at meals. A nibble that would have been a part of a meal does not add to the total intake—it simply is eaten at a slightly different time of day. As you suggested, it also is helpful to keep busy with work, hobbies, or physical activity. Since many people eat to relieve boredom, such activities certainly may be helpful in preventing and treating overweight.

What is the caloric content of buttermilk in comparison with skim or nonfat milk? What other comparisons can be made between dairy products?

Buttermilk and nonfat or skim milk have about the same calorie content. Although buttermilk is not often mentioned on reducing menus, don't hesitate to substitute it for the skim milk in the plan. This is an interesting way of adding some variety to the diet. The caloric contribution of the various commercial cottage cheeses varies, but the uncreamed types average about 26–30 calories per ounce, while the creamed cottage cheeses are somewhat higher, ranging from 30 to 35 calories per ounce.

And now here's your chance to find out what you know about weight control. Test your knowledge by taking this test.

WEIGHT CONTROL QUIZ

When you look at Mrs. Five-by-Five, obesity seems as clear as the nose on her face, or the fat on her waist. Yet obesity is like an iceberg; there's more to it than appears on the surface. Some of these hidden facts are still mysterious; they baffle the experts who try to explain obesity and also the sufferers who try to overcome it. Yet, even without knowing the full extent of icebergs, navigators have the sense to try to avoid them. And experts know enough about obesity to be sure it too is dangerous and should be avoided. How many of these facts do you know?

1. Obesity is the enemy of longevity. If a person is obese, the chances for a long and healthy life decrease by a. 79%, b. 42%, c. 10%
2. What relation does obesity have to, a. Diabetes?, b. Hypertension and heart disease?
3. Which of the following statements is accurate: a. Increased activity burns extra calories and therefore helps weight loss, b. Decreased activity is advisable because it cuts down appetite.

4. Which system is the weight loser's best bet? a. A combination of decreased food intake and increased activity, b. A diet low in carbohydrate with unlimited fat and calories, or c. Total or semi-starvation, with an assist from a "reducing" drug.

5. How much is enough weight for a healthy adult? a. Are 152 or 165 pounds an appropriate weight for a 40-year-old man who is 5'10" tall?, b. Are 108 or 138 pounds an appropriate weight for a 40-year-old women who is 5'4" tall?

6. How much is enough for an adult's daily intake of kilocalories? a. Are 1,800 or 2,500 calories enough for a women?, b. Are 2,000 or 3,000 calories enough for a man?

7. How much is enough exercise? a. To burn up the 150 calories in ½-cup of ordinary ice cream or a cocktail or highball?, b. For fitness in a healthy adult?

And now for the answers:

1. If your answer is c, you are an optimist. Either a or b is correct, depending upon the degree of overweight. Even moderate obesity increases the chance of mortality by 42%, according to Drs. Hashim and Van Itallie, former members of Harvard's Department of Nutrition and now at the Obesity Clinic of St. Lukes Hospital in New York City. Markedly overweight persons decrease their chance of enjoying a full life span (and more years of good eating) by 79%.

2. Obesity is a complication in diabetes, hypertension, and heart disease. Just think—90% of patients who become diabetic after age 30 are overweight! Hypertension and heart disease also are definitely aggravated by the burden which extra pounds impose on the heart and other organs.

3. Any argument against activity is a convenient alibi for the lazy, but false. A is 100% correct. Activity requires energy, and if this isn't being supplied by foods, it will come from body fat. That's how exercise—if it's regular—can make a sizable dent in body weight.

4. What's your goal? If you want to stun your friends and fit into a new outfit for a night, most anything can be successful. Temporary starvation or fad diets or high-powered reducing drugs will all help to take off the weight, but briefly. This kind of slimness never, never lasts. There is just one sure way if you want to wear that new outfit after six months or a year. Overweight is only overcome by a combination of moderate diet and moderate exercise that can be followed for weeks, months, and years. This system has no competitor for long-term success.

5. The weight that is enough for an adult is the average weight for people of that sex and height at age 25. Statistics show that the individuals who keep that weight, which is called Desirable Weight, live longer, stay healthier in the process, and are less apt to have heart attacks and many other diseases than those who go on gaining. Therefore, it doesn't matter whether the man or woman in our question is 40, 30, or 70. After 25, the 5'10" man should always maintain his weight in the range between 152 and 165 pounds, depending upon his frame and muscles. Similarly, the 5'4" woman should weigh somewhere between 108 pounds for a small frame and 138 pounds for a large frame and should stay that way forever and ever.

6. The moderately active woman whose Desirable Weight is 128 pounds probably requires about 2,200 calories daily at age 25, 1,850 at 45, and 1,700 at age 65. The moderately active man weighing 154 pounds needs approximately 2,800 calories daily at age 25, 2,600 at age 45, and 2,400 at age 65. In other words, *energy intake* (from food and drink) MUST be decreased when age goes up because work (exercise and energy expenditure) usually goes down.

7. Remember that many factors affect energy expenditure. In general, however, one can burn up 150 calories by bicycling or playing tennis or sawing wood for 20–30 minutes, by spending half an hour at vigorous housework or walking briskly, or by typing or washing dishes for about 1½ hours. The answer to part *b* is that many people definitely are not active enough either to burn up the extra calories they consume or to keep their bodies fit. That is why regular exercise is necessary. How much? Thirty minutes daily is not too much and 15 is better than none! Who is there who cannot adjust a busy schedule to include at least two 15-minute periods of brisk physical activity, such as walking at a good clip, if it will help health and longevity?

And last but not least, indeed perhaps most important, is *portion size*. Two pieces of bread have twice the calories of one piece; six ounces of steak have twice the calories of three ounces; a martini with three ounces of gin has twice the calories of one with half that amount of gin—and so on and so on.

This simple concept of portion size led one of us (FJS) many years ago to coin the phrase that "cutting down, not out, with a little cutting up" is the secret of weight control. And by cutting up is meant more physical activity.

One can really have any food or drink, depending on portion size on a reducing diet, but the portion sizes must be small enough so that in any and every 24-hour period the total calories consumed must be fewer than those expended. If this is the case, then to provide those extra calories expended one has to draw upon stored body energy (fat deposits) and weight will be lost.

Forget about all the "odd ball diets, such as the Beverly Hills Diet, the I Love New York Diet, the low carbohydrate, high fiber, high protein, etc., diets, and eat a well balanced diet made up of foods you enjoy, but *keep portion sizes down.*

2

THE "HEARTY" EATER AND OTHER HEALTH PROBLEMS

Cardiovascular diseases are the leading cause of death in this country, claiming more than 900,000 lives each year. Coronary heart disease is the major cardiovascular disease. For years, we have known that a high blood cholesterol level may increase one's chances of suffering from coronary heart disease (CHD).

The direct cause of CHD also has been well documented for many years. The blood supply to the heart muscle is blocked by deposits of cholesterol, a waxy substance produced in the liver and also acquired from outside in certain foods, especially egg yolks, animal fats, and milk products. These blockages develop chiefly because the cholesterol level in the blood is too high and it sets up deposits in the arteries (atherosclerosis), which ultimately cause trouble by narrowing the blood vessels. The narrowed vessel may become completely blocked by a blood clot.

However, the science of cholesterol is getting increasingly sophisticated. We now realize that there are different types of "carriers" for cholesterol, classified according to their size and density. There is now very convincing evidence from studies of human populations that one type of lipoprotein known as alpha-cholesterol or High Density Lipoprotein (HDL) may actually protect us from heart disease, while another type, beta-cholesterol or Low Density Lipoprotein (LDL), can significantly increase chances of developing serious heart troubles.

Reports from a 26-year-old research program funded by the National Heart, Lung, and Blood Institute, indicate that individuals with low levels of HDL have eight times or more greater incidence of heart disease than do those with relatively higher levels of HDL. This finding, which has been confirmed in studies around the world, helps explain a few of the somewhat puzzling observations noted about the frequency of CHD. It is consistent with observations about who is and who is not likely to be a victim of CHD.

For example, it has been known for decades that women in their reproductive years have a much lower rate of heart disease than do men of a similar age. It has now been shown that women in this age group have 30 to 60 percent more HDL than do their male counterparts. (Studies in laboratories also indicate that the HDL levels of dogs and rats, species quite resistant to atherosclerosis, are very high.) Diabetics, obese individuals, and those with high blood pressure all have a high risk of heart disease and all have low levels of HDL. Cigarette smokers, who also have a high risk of heart disease, do not have significantly lower HDL levels. This suggests that the way smoking affects heart health may be different from the way these other risk factors do. And an enigma which has long intrigued public health specialists has now been explained. Eskimos, as a population group, have high serum cholesterol levels, mostly as HDL, but a low rate of coronary heart disease.

How exactly HDL in the blood protects us from heart disease is not fully established, but it is thought that this lipoprotein serves to carry protein which helps the removal of cholesterol from the tissues to the liver and blocks the tissues from aiding the transport of the LDL.

Now that the concept of "blood cholesterol" has been broken down into types, and "good cholesterol" can be distinguished from "bad cholesterol," the question is to how to apply this knowledge for better heart health.

As of now, all the answers are not in, but at least one point is clear. The goal is not to get rid of cholesterol completely, for cholesterol is a necessary substance in our bodies. It is important in the repair of ruptured membranes, in the production of sex hormones and vitamin D, and in making bile acids. The idea is to keep your overall cholesterol level at a reasonable figure and to keep the HDL level, in particular, as high as possible.

Two possible means of influencing total cholesterol and HDL levels are now being recommended. First, for many people, diet can play a major role in controlling cholesterol production. We now have preliminary evidence indicating that not only does a diet low in cholesterol and saturated fats depress total cholesterol levels, but it is likely to increase the HDL level. It has been shown, for example, that the HDL levels among vegetarians are consistently and significantly higher than those of meat eaters. We are not suggesting that you give up meat (unless you choose to). However, you should be sensible about eating a balanced diet, taking the most logical approach to stopping the deposits of cholesterol in the coronary arteries by modifying the typical American overly rich diet. Use more *lean meat*, and drain the fat from meat you have cooked. Eat more fruits, vegetables, and cereal products, and limit your consumption of egg yolks (the whites are excellent protein sources with no cholesterol) to 3 or 4 per week. Use skim or lowfat dairy products instead of those made with whole milk.

Exercise is another possible way of increasing HDL levels. It is unclear whether it is exercise per se which has an advantageous effect on lipoproteins, or if it is the resulting effect that exercise has on keeping weight down, and thus controlling blood pressure. A study at Louisiana State University Medical School showed that, when students participated in exercise programs of four daily 30-minute, intense physical exercise periods a week, their HDL levels increased significantly. Similarly, a research team from the Stanford Heart Disease Prevention Program compared fasting plasma and lipoprotein levels of 41 male long distance runners, aged 35–59, with a randomly selected group of men of a comparable age. All the runners had registered at least 15 miles a week in the previous year—so they were not exactly casual exercisers.

The team noted that the HDL levels in the runners were significantly higher than in the control group, and concluded,

> These very active men exhibited a plasma lipoprotein profile resembling that of younger women rather than of sedentary middle-aged men. This characteristic and apparently advantageous pattern could only partially be accounted for by differences in (body weight) between runners and control subjects.

How do you do your best to ensure good heart health? Our advice is simple and straightforward: Have your cholesterol level and your HDL and LDL levels checked during your annual physical (any laboratory that can perform a serum cholesterol determination can perform an HDL and LDL cholesterol determination if what is known as a refrigerated centrifuge is available). Be aware of the risk factors (too many total calories and saturated fat and cholesterol-rich diets, lack of exercise, cigarette smoking, obesity, diabetes, high blood pressure) and modify your lifestyle to minimize these risks.

A GLOBAL VIEW OF CHOLESTEROL

Because heart disease remains such a serious public health problem in the United States, even though deaths from it have decreased some 20% in the past decade, it continues to be the subject of a great deal of study. Many scientists have sought clues to causes by comparing Americans with groups in other countries. One suggestion has been that our "national diet" is at fault, that there is some connection in American men between their high saturated fat diets, their high blood cholesterol levels, and their susceptibility to heart disease.

This brings up an interesting question: what happens to other people in other parts of the world who also consume large amounts of milk and meat? Some revealing observations on this were reported a few years ago by Dr. George Mann, formerly of Harvard's Department of Nutrition and now at Vanderbilt University. He had planned to study the Eskimos, since they once belonged to the category of meat eaters. This proved unsatisfactory, for they no longer adhere to their ancestral traditions in diet.

For the Congo Pygmies, however, meat is still the mainstay of the diet. Despite this, Dr. Mann found that the men had the lowest blood cholesterol levels yet recorded for men anywhere in the world.

Dr. Mann also studied the Masai in Africa, and they proved to be particularly interesting from a dietary point of view. From their "initiation" at the age of 15 to their marriage some 20 years later, these warriors live mainly on meat and milk. How do they spend their time? They scorn farming and devote themselves to caring for their prized cattle. For diversion, the men hunt lions and the other wild animals which threaten their families and their herds. Both of these pursuits require endless walking and running.

The Masai are lean and tall, with excellent teeth. Unfortunately, they suffer from many infections, especially malaria, intestinal parasites, venereal disease, and tuberculosis, but they have low blood pressure and far less evidence of heart disease than American men of comparable ages.

Why are the Masai comparatively free of heart disease? One possible explanation is that these men are protected by the exercise they get regularly in their daily lives. Americans sit at desks, in front of the television, in cars, and in golf carts. The Masai move, and they don't use cars, elevators, trolleys, buses, or planes to do it. For the Masai, it's footwork every step of the way, for countless miles of travel.

Does this activity make the difference? Does this keep the Masai lean, and does that help? Or are they born with an extra something that protects them? Perhaps it is the simple life that saves the Masai from heart trouble. American men eat and drink too much, do not get enough exercise, and may have too many worries and frustrations.

No one is certain. Until we can be sure, perhaps there is a lesson the Masai can teach us. We can't indulge in lion hunting every day, but we can move more than we do, and we can stay slim. Moderate eating and moderate exercising won't accomplish miracles, but many people agree that they are important steps in the right direction.

EXERCISE AND HEART ATTACKS

Does exercise play any part in the prevention of heart attacks? Is it valuable, harmful, or unimportant?

Evidence regarding the value of exercise has been coming into focus gradually as historical information and current research studies are assessed in relation to the incidence of heart disease. For instance, in England some years ago it was found that motormen had more heart attacks than conductors. Why? A very good reason seemed to be that the motormen sat at their jobs all day, whereas the conductors spent their working hours running up and down the stairs of their big double-decker buses.

Equally striking is evidence from Israel which suggests similar conclusions. A few years ago a 10-year study was conducted in 58 kibbutz settlements which included 4,500 men and 4,000 women, ranging between ages 30 and 55 at the beginning of the study. Records were available giving complete information about the job history and health record of all of these participants.

The kibbutz pattern of living lends itself very well to dietary studies because food, clothes, housing, and all other necessities are provided on a share-and-share-alike basis. Everyone works according to age and ability and receives according to need. Adults live in their own rooms, with children being housed in separate quarters and under the supervision of specially trained personnel. All are served by a communal kitchen. This makes it possible to regulate, check, and calculate food intake.

As a result of the general physical layout of the kibbutz, everyone received about the same amount of physical exercise from walking between the home area and work, and the dining hall. The primary variable was the type of work that the various people did. This turned out to be a very significant variable! The incidence of heart attacks was three times greater among the sedentary men than among those engaged in active physical labor. Among the women, the sedentary workers had five times more heart attacks than those who were assigned physically active jobs.

These findings bear out other observations that physical activity may help prevent heart attacks. Perhaps the many mechanical devices in our world today may be desirable as labor savers, but not as heart savers.

Heart disease has aroused attention among research scientists and practicing physicians in the United States, but the interest does not stop there.

FREQUENTLY ASKED QUESTIONS ABOUT HEART DISEASE

A man in Maryland writes that he is 40 years old and has a good wife, a happy life, and four children to support and educate. He is worried because he knows several middle-aged people who have had heart attacks, and he wants to do what he can to avoid having this happen to him.

In response to this query, there definitely are risk factors that are significant in heart disease, and it is certainly wise to pay attention to these. No one can guarantee that any one individual will be sure of avoiding an attack, but often preventive care proves to be of crucial importance. The chances are definitely better, both for prevention of and recovery from heart attacks, if an individual maintains desirable weight, cuts out cigarettes, exercises regularly, and attempts to control any associated diseases, particularly an increase in blood pressure, even if only a slight increase. All of us, no matter how robust we think we are, can greatly improve our health and longevity if we follow two essential courses of action: (1) see a doctor for regular physical checkups (and these should include a measurement of blood pressure and blood cholesterol), and (2) establish good eating, exercise, and living habits, which include reaching and maintaining desirable weight, no smoking, and adequate rest.

A man in California inquires whether he needs to reduce if he wants to minimize his likelihood for having a heart attack. He points out that there is no heart disease in his family, but he is overweight.

Certainly it is a greater likelihood that a person with a combination of predisposing factors (including a family history of heart or vascular disease early in life, before age 60) will have a heart attack sooner than the person who has none of these factors working against him. However, other abnormalities, such as diabetes, hypothyroidism, and kidney trouble are also significant. Unfortunately, according to a report presented at a recent national conference on cardiovascular diseases, there are few low risk middle-aged men in our population. The majority have two or even three risk factors. And even if you do not fit into these groups, you should remember that obesity is a complication or risk factor not only in coronary heart disease, but also in other medical conditions. What's more, obese people who reduce their weight increase their chances of avoiding a heart attack or of recovering if they have one. So our answer to you is, "Yes, you should reduce, and don't put it off until tomorrow!"

With all this emphasis on exercise, it's not surprising that the question arises as to what kind of exercise is recommended for people in their 50s.

Of course, practically all kinds of exercise are good and valuable when they are done on a reasonably regular basis and are geared to one's individual capacity. Exercise need not, and indeed should not, be too strenuous; what is most important is that it should be regular. One half-hour every day is a good goal, and this can be in two 15-minute periods. We hope the future will see much more cooperation on this score between the community and the individual. What can the community do? Construction of bicycle paths, hiking trails, and golf courses, provision of swimming facilities, gyms, tennis courts, and areas for active recreation in new housing developments and older neighborhoods are appropriate community goals. The individual can aid by stimulating public interest in such developments, making use of existing facilities, and getting in the habit of doing a little vigorous exercise which causes huffing and puffing.

To the person who has heart disease, there are three major guidelines:

1. Avoid overweight, and if overweight start now to get it down, gradually but surely. This is important regardless of the kind of heart disease. Calorie input and energy output need to be balanced carefully by close cooperation between patient and physician. Improper dieting may be not only ineffective, but possibly harmful.
2. Avoid foods and situations that cause trouble. Don't eat foods you know disagree with you. Don't eat too much at one time. In some kinds of heart trouble, an over-loaded stomach puts an undesirable extra burden on the heart. Finally, don't eat when you are nervous, upset, or rushed.

3. Follow your diet. If your physician has prescribed a diet, it is an important part of your *treatment*. Be sure to follow your own diet that the doctor or the dietitian has prescribed specifically for your condition. Be sure to ask questions if there are aspects of the diet program that you do not understand.

JAWBREAKERS

The vocabulary used to talk about the nutritional factors that may influence coronary heart disease is meaningful to a scientist, but is likely to seem mysterious and alarming to the non-scientist. By now, we have all become accustomed to seeing ads in magazines and newspapers describing the virtues of "polyunsaturated" vegetable oils. We have even managed to learn to pronounce cholesterol without stumbling over it, but just what do these terms mean to your general health?

It may come as a surprise to you that cholesterol is an organic compound that is normally found in the body. This substance is actually needed by the body for several important functions. For example, vitamin D is formed in your skin from cholesterol and similar compounds when you are exposed to sunlight. Cholesterol also is used to form some of the sex hormones. It is apparent that cholesterol in the body is necessary and normal. The concern about cholesterol is that increased cholesterol levels in the blood often are found in patients with coronary heart disease. Because of this relationship between increased blood cholesterol and coronary heart disease, there has been a great deal of research by nutrition scientists to determine whether diet controls blood cholesterol levels. It has been found that diet is an important factor, but not the only one that determines your blood cholesterol level. This is where all the confusing information about fats and polyunsaturates comes into play.

The basic chemistry of fats has been known for quite a long time. Even without any knowledge of chemistry, it is obvious that the type of fat varies from one kind of animal to another. Beef fat characteristically is considerably harder than pork fat, for example. And all animal fats are definitely firmer than the oils that are extracted from peanuts, olives, corn, and other vegetable sources. The harder animal fats are slightly different chemically from most of the vegetable oils because they contain more hydrogen. Fatty substances containing all the hydrogen they can chemically hold are saturated fats. Animal fats are comparatively good sources of these saturated fats. But there are at least two exceptions—coconut and palm oils, certainly not animal fats, are very high in saturated fats. The oils from peanuts and olives could hold just a bit more hydrogen, and so they are said to be monounsaturated. The oils from corn, soybeans, cottonseed, safflower, and sunflower seeds can hold still more hydrogen; they are said to be polyunsaturated.

Evidence indicates that the saturated fats from meats encourage a rise in your blood cholesterol level, particularly if one is overweight, and that the oils that can hold more hydrogen will help to lower your blood cholesterol level. Now, don't immediately assume that this means you should eliminate meat from your diet! You need it for its protein, iron, vitamin and trace mineral content. However, it does mean that you would be wise to cut off the visible fat in meat rather than eat it. It also means that you should cut down the *size* of your meat servings (portion size) to three or four ounces of cooked meat. You may wish to begin eating more poultry and fish, for these are types of meat that are relatively low in total fat, particularly saturated fats. You will find that margarines made from corn, soybean, cottonseed, sunflower, or safflower oils are acceptable to you, and these are high in polyunsaturates. It is generally a good idea for overweight people to reduce the amount of saturated fat in the diet and replace some of it with polyunsaturated fats.

When we recommend an increase in polyunsaturated fats in the diet (in place of some of the saturated fats) as one of the nutritional procedures to help lower blood cholesterol, we are not recommending "wallowing" in oils loaded with linoleic acid. Rather, we are suggesting that instead of diets providing 3 to 4% of total calories from polyunsaturated fats, they provide 8 to 10%. This can readily be accomplished by using polyunsaturated margarine in place of butter, using cooking and salad oils higher in polyunsaturates and lower in saturates, and using more chicken and fish in place of some of the meat.

It is easy to recommend dietary changes, but to change dietary habits is indeed an awesome task.

CHANGING DIETARY HABITS

Can adults in this country be persuaded to modify their diets? They certainly can, and two striking examples are the generous use of orange and tomato juice during the past few decades.

Man has always been interested in health, his own health, and the older he gets, the more interest he has in health. The development of nutrition as a science (the science of food in relation to health), has motivated the public to be far more aware of the influence of food on health. This is particularly true in recent years because of the influence nutrition has had on speeding up or retarding the development of our commonest cause of death, coronary heart disease.

A few years ago, our laboratory at Harvard and four other medical centers completed the first stage of one of the world's more extensive studies in which the effectiveness of lessening risk factors in reducing coronary heart disease was measured. The risk factors being evaluated were blood pressure, blood cholesterol, body weight, and cigarette smoking. The question being answered is whether men living in a free society will limit themselves to the diet on which they have been instructed if they think it might lessen their chance of having a heart attack.

The diet was restricted in eggs and contained specially prepared foods in which the fats had been modified in quantity and quality. In many cases, these foods did not taste familiar, and the volunteers had to forego the pleasure of bacon, marbled beef, and thick lamb chops. Would they eat this different food and be happy? The answer was definitely *yes*. In fact, less than 10 percent of the men withdrew from the program, and the reasons for withdrawal were generally because of family situations, travel commitments, or change of position, and not because of the food. The men were remarkably loyal to the diet and to keeping their many appointments at the clinic. Most of the wives were equally enthusiastic about the diet and were cooperative.

The effects of these foods on the level of cholesterol in the body and on body weight were as expected—decreases. The findings indicate that it is safe to conclude that men will eat new foods, reduce intake of certain foods, and adhere to a new diet if properly motivated.

With the completion of this study, which involved only changes in diet, a new and larger study is currently in progress. The new study concerns not only diet changes but changes in smoking, exercise, and other functions thought to affect susceptibility to heart disease. It is underway in some 20 centers around the country, including Harvard's Department of Nutrition. The results should be available in 1983.

BEVERAGES AND YOUR HEART

Certainly beverages are a part of any person's diet, whether heart disease is in the picture or not. Therefore, it is wise to consider just what the possible and probable effects of common beverages are.

Because of the caffeine in coffee, the question is sometimes asked whether coffee is harmful and should be avoided by those who are prone to heart disease or who already have it. Present knowledge indicates that it is all right for people with heart problems to drink some coffee, but with some qualifications.

Anything is harmful when consumed to excess, even water. Coffee does have some caffeine, which is a stimulant. This is why many of us like coffee in the morning to help us get going. There are a few people who are unusually sensitive to caffeine and in these, one or two cups will cause a jittery feeling. In some people who have varying degrees of high blood pressure, it may be that coffee causes a further increase in the blood pressure. Obviously, such individuals should not consume coffee, or at least should consume it in smaller amounts than produce such results.

There have been reports in the medical literature of a positive association or relationship between those who drink more than six or eight cups of coffee per day and those who have had heart attacks. However, it is likely that these individuals were also overweight, had higher levels of cholesterol in the blood, elevated blood pressure, were heavy cigarette smokers, etc., so just coffee could not really be blamed as the culprit. So as far as we know, coffee is a pleasant beverage and can be consumed by most individuals at levels varying up to six or eight cups a day without any known hazard to health. In fact, coffee is a good source of niacin, one of the B vitamins.

A senior citizen with angina pectoris asks whether alcoholic beverages are good for him because he had heard that alcohol dilates the arteries. Angina pectoris, or pain in the chest, is a common symptom due to narrowing of the coronary arteries, the vessels which supply blood to the heart muscle. The standard treatment is nitroglycerine put under the tongue. Evaluation and treatment of angina should be made by a physician, not by the individual or friends. Nitroglycerine tablets dilate the blood vessels of the heart and permit better blood circulation in that vital organ. Alcohol dilates blood vessels throughout the body, including the blood vessels of the heart. It is a fact that patients with angina may derive comfort from a drink containing alcohol. Many physicians recommend two or three ounces of brandy, whiskey, or gin in the late afternoon or evening for individuals who are bothered with angina. This is effective largely because of inducing some relaxation from the tensions of the day. Wine or other alcoholic beverages may be equally effective.

TIPS ON FOODS FOR CHOLESTEROL FIGHTERS

By now you are well aware of the need to control your weight, to stop smoking, and to exercise on a daily basis as three ways of maintaining optimum health. In addition, some attention to the intake of foods high in cholesterol and saturated fats, particularly if you are overweight, and to including some polyunsaturated vegetable oil in place of some of the saturated fats will help to keep your cholesterol within the desirable range. If you tend toward hypercholesterolemia (high blood cholesterol levels), you should restrict your intake of egg yolks to only two or three per week and substitute polyunsaturated fats (corn, sunflower, safflower, cottonseed, or soya oil or their products) for much of the saturated fats (butter and meat fats) you now consume. Fish and poultry are good foods to eat more frequently than you probably do now. Their calorie content is lower than red meats because of their lower fat content, and the fat they contain is less saturated than animal fats.

You will want to consume shellfish sparingly, for some are rather high in cholesterol. Lobster and shrimp are the highest, with levels in the range of 135–180 milligrams (mg) per three ounces; clams, oysters, crabs, and scallops have less cholesterol, but still somewhat more than ordinary fish or meat. Organ meats such as liver contain more cholesterol than muscle meats. For comparative figures, one egg yolk provides 250 to 300 mg, three ounces of roast beef contain 70 to 90 mg, a like amount of liver has 300–320 mg, and a 6-ounce glass of milk has 20 mg of cholesterol in it. Thus, we feel that eggs (only the yolks contain cholesterol), liver or shellfish can be used once or twice a week, but should not be a frequent part of the diet of people with elevated cholesterol levels.

Another dietary problem is the habit of salting all food generously, even when it has not yet been tasted. Using less salt is a desirable food habit to develop.

ASSAULT ON SALT

There has been considerable concern recently about the amount of salt in the diet and its relationship to hypertension, or high blood pressure. There are an estimated 30 to 40 million cases of hypertension in the United States alone, and an estimated 20 percent of the world population is afflicted. Yet research done in 1976 indicated that in about 90 percent of the cases studied, no actual cause of hypertension could be determined.

The possible role of salt (specifically the sodium ion) in hypertension has been under careful study for some 60 years, but it still is not generally accepted that sodium causes hypertension. It has been known, though, that the blood pressure of many unmedicated patients with hypertension will go down when the sodium in their diets is drastically restricted (below half a gram per day). It is also known that their blood pressure will increase again when substantial amounts of sodium are returned to their diets. However, blood pressure in about 80% of people does not increase even though they consumed sodium far in excess of the small amounts needed (0.5 to 1.0 gram per day).

A positive relationship between the estimated average amount of salt consumed and hypertension has been concluded by many (but not all) studies of various ethnic populations. However, these are non-specific epidemiological studies, and often cannot specify other possible correlating causes of hypertension, such as genetic predisposition, obesity, general nutritional status, and potassium intake. It has also been impossible to study carefully enough the differences among individuals of various cultures.

Since the sodium ion is known to play a major role in regulating body fluids, we can assume that it is capable of influencing blood pressure, whether or not it actually causes hypertension. For this reason, we advise everyone, certainly those who are otherwise at risk for high blood pressure, to resist the automatic impulse to sprinkle a little more salt on everything, and to limit dietary salt by cutting down on the amount of extra-salty snacks. However, salt must not be considered a total "badditive." It is an essential part of the human diet.

In the midst of the current worry about salt, it is important to recognize its physiological value to man and all mammals. We would be most unhealthy and unhappy were we to become salt-deficient. In fact, we would be subject to headaches, weakness, giddiness, lack of concentration, poor memory, and poor appetite, as well as find our food unbearably unpleasant if this were to happen.

Table salt actually is sodium chloride. When dissolved in water, it separates into two ions—one of sodium and one of chloride. The sodium ion is required for maintaining the pressure and volume of blood. It also is essential in controlling the passage of water into and out of the body's cells, and the relative volumes of fluids inside and outside those cells also are influenced by sodium. The sodium ion is necessary for transmitting nerve impulses and for metabolizing carbohydrates and proteins.

The chloride ion is essential for maintaining the acid-base balance in the blood, and for the passage of water across cell walls to maintain proper concentrations of various chemicals. It is needed for activating certain enzymes and for forming hydrochloric acid in the stomach for food digestion.

Both sodium and chloride must be provided in the diet. It has been difficult to determine exactly what amounts are required by humans, but the most frequent estimate of the minimum daily adult requirement is 200 mg of sodium (0.5 grams of salt). However, no known national diets commonly contain such small amounts of salt.

For most American consumers today, such a diet would seem very dull, even unpalatable, in view of the fact that their total daily intake of salt ranges from 10 to 12 grams (3,900 to 4,700 mg of sodium) or somewhat more. These figures include about three grams of salt occurring naturally in the food eaten, three grams added by the cook and at the table, plus some four to six grams added during commercial processing of food.

Because there is such variability as to how individuals use the salt shaker and nibble on salty snacks, or use other sodium-containing foods like soy sauce and monosodium glutamate (MSG), it is impossible to be precise with estimates of amounts actually used. (It should be pointed out that because of the difference in molecular weight, MSG contains about half the amount of sodium as does salt.)

Individual salt requirements fluctuate also, depending on several factors: amount and intensity of physical activity, the quantity and composition of sweat, environmental conditions, and weather conditions. Since it is impossible to calculate how much salt is lost in sweating at different temperatures and activities, determining how much is necessary to replace it is also impossible. Salt deficiency is not likely to occur among Americans, because most tend to consume far greater amounts than are required physiologically, with the palate serving as a safeguard.

When there is a high intake of salt, sodium and chloride are not normally stored in the body. The excess amounts are excreted, so that the sodium level in the body is maintained within very narrow limits, as is chloride, regardless of the intake. Substantial amounts are lost in sweat and the feces, but the primary route of excretion is via the urine. The fact that the normal body does not store sodium and chloride is interesting in view of the fact that the normal body does not reveal increased blood pressure when fed excessive amounts of sodium.

Sodium compounds occur naturally in many foods, including meats, fish, dairy products, and vegetables. Even drinking water, especially from deep wells, contains sodium in varying amounts, whether or not the water is softened. Softened water contains generous amounts of sodium because a sodium-containing chemical is used in the softening process.

For centuries, salt has been widely used as a preservative, and it is essential for processing meats and cheese products. By controlling certain microorganisms, it allows sauerkraut to "emerge" from shredded cabbage, and different kinds of cheeses to form from identical dairy cultures. It also controls texture and moisture levels in many foods—all the while adding its own pleasant flavor.

The microbiological stability of a given food, its likelihood of spoilage, also depends on its water activity. Each microorganism has a value for water activity, above which it will grow and below which it will not. Some foods are dried or dehydrated to reduce water activity, and sometimes hydrophilic ("water-loving") chemicals are added, as in certain meat and cheese products.

Because salt is one of the most effective agents for lowering water activity, it is often used to alter the environment within a food so that the growth of undesirable organisms is retarded or prevented, and the growth of desirable ones is encouraged.

For example, in the production of sauerkraut, pickles, fermented sausages, and cheese, salt is used to withdraw water and various nutrients from the tissue, thus providing the proper environment for growing the desirable bacteria. The undesirable microorganisms that would cause spoilage are also controlled by the salt. The accumulation of organic acids formed during fermentation can then be controlled by the desirable microorganisms and processes that exclude oxygen. If too much salt is used, desirable fermentation will be delayed, while too little salt will result in poor quality or product loss due to undesirable fermentation.

In making cheese, adding salt to the milled curd after cheddaring helps to remove the whey, suppress the growth of undesirable microorganisms, slow down acid development, and produce the desired flavor. If too much salt is added, the cheese will be dry and brittle, while too little salt will cause it to have a weak and pasty body.

High levels of salt can be put in cheese curd to inhibit most of the microorganisms but allow the mold, *Pennicillium roqueforti,* to grow and produce blue cheese. Or, certain bacteria may be added to lightly-salted cheese curd to create the "eyes" and sweet flavor of the Swiss cheeses. The dehydrating effect of salt also helps to form the rind of cheeses.

In canned vegetables, the heat processing provides the preserving action, so salt is added primarily for flavoring. Frozen vegetables, with the exception of lima beans, butter beans, mixed vegetables, and peas, usually do not have added salt. Nor is salt generally used in the processing of fruits for freezing or canning.

In the case of lima beans, butter beans, mixed vegetables, and peas, a salt brine often is used to separate the overly mature vegetables from the younger ones. The younger ones will float while the older ones sink. The sorted beans and peas are then washed with water before freezing. Some vegetables and fruits have their peels removed by being passed through a hot lye (sodium hydroxide) bath, after which they are washed. Residual sodium from both of these processes is very low.

The average amount of salt added to canned vegetables is from 0.6 per cent to 1 percent of the finished product (undrained), but the amounts vary with specific vegetables. Canned whole-kernel corn may have about 255 mg of salt per 100 grams of corn; and canned green beans may have as much as 380 mg of salt per 100 grams of beans.

Salt (sodium) content of processed meats is extremely variable and often considerably higher than that of the raw product. For instance, fresh pork sausage may contain as little as ¾ percent sodium, while dried chipped beef may contain as much as 4.35 percent sodium or almost 11 percent salt. Country ham processed in the traditional way may contain up to 3 percent sodium. Most processed meats contain between 1.1 and 1.3 percent sodium, but no really reliable average is available.

Salt brine contributes most of the added sodium in the 200-odd cured meat and sausage items on the market. However, curing ingredients such as sodium nitrite, used as a preservative against deadly botulism and to provide the "cured" taste and pink color, contribute varying amounts of sodium. Sodium phosphates, often used in cured meats to reduce shrinkage during processing and to retard rancidity, also contribute to the total sodium content.

Nonfat dry milk is sometimes added to processed meats as a non-meat protein to supplement the binding effect of the salt-soluble meat protein. This can contain from 535 to 2,280 mg of sodium per 100 grams of meat. Whey-derived products, soy-derived protein additives, hydrolyzed vegetable protein, and monosodium glutamate all contain sodium, and all are additives allowed by the government, in relatively low levels, in different products. Meat fiber itself contains sodium—about 55 mg per 100 grams in beef, and 65 mg per 100 grams in pork.

The level of sodium in wheat flours is quite low (2 to 3 mg per 100 grams). However, most finished bakery and other grain products contain considerably larger amounts. Added salt is the primary source of sodium, but baking soda and certain leavening acids contribute sodium, too. Three slices of bread contain about 1 gram of salt (400 mg of sodium).

Salt is added to bakery products mainly for flavor. It has a way of enhancing other flavors in a product. But it has other significant roles, most important being control of the rate of fermentation of yeast-leavened products. Salt controls the growth rate of desirable microorganisms and prevents the development of undesirable, uncontrollable types of yeast which would spoil the fermentation process. In addition, salt reduces the water-absorption rate of the dough and has a strengthening effect on the gluten which helps make dough easier to handle.

Baking soda, with or without various leavening acids, is another source of sodium in the diet. Calcium and sodium phosphates are the most widely used leavening agents, and they contain sodium. Less sodium is found in sodium aluminum phosphates, which have become popular in recent years as a leavening agent.

For people on salt-restricted diets, there are salt-free breads available, but they have not been popular. Foods such as pretzels, potato chips, and popcorn often are heavily salted purely for flavor, and these are the foods we recommend restricting first when you have to cut down on salt consumption. For many people, eliminating these foods is more pleasant than resorting to unsalted bread.

Very few prescription drugs contain sodium, but the non-prescription, over-the-counter drugs do. Some antacids can supply a total daily sodium intake of 1,200 mg (3 grams of salt), or as much as 7,000 mg, but most are in the range of 100 to 200 mg of sodium a day. For instance, aspirin contains 49 mg per dose, and in fact, this can cause trouble for people on salt-restricted diets. But the antacid pain relievers, laxatives, and sleep aids which combine sodium-containing antacids are even more worrisome. Bromo-Seltzer contains 717 mg per dose, and Alka-Seltzer contains 521 mg per dose. The antacid laxative Sal Hepatica contains three sodium compounds and yields 1,000 mg of sodium per dose!

If sodium restriction is necessary, be sure to scan all labels carefully and to consult your physician or a health professional about the sodium content of the various products and the potential danger to you.

The ratio of potassium to sodium in the body is very important and should be considered when evaluating diets. Some studies have shown that increased intake of potassium chloride can reduce blood pressure in hypertensive patients, even in the presence of excess sodium chloride. A mixture of sodium and potassium chloride for "salting" food may benefit people with hypertension. A ratio of 1 to 1 will not produce a noticeable change in taste for most people, and exclusive use of such a mixture could eliminate as much as 1½ grams of salt daily from the average diet. Excessive amounts of potassium chloride should be avoided, however, because of toxicity at very high levels.

The decisions about which sources of salt to restrict are yours. We hope we've helped you to make them intelligently. In case you would still like a bit more insight into the problem of sodium, read on.

Are salt requirements and tolerances the same for all people?

No. Salt requirements and tolerances are specific for each individual. The potential hazard in consuming too much salt is also specific for each individual, depending on factors such as general health, genetic vulnerability, stress, and obesity.

Should everyone cut down on salted foods?

Not necessarily. However, since approximately 20 percent of the world population is potentially sensitive to salt (specifically, sodium), we think it is important for everyone to be aware of salt sources and uses in order to determine whether or not they are consuming too much salt, and if so, what sources can readily be reduced to decrease the quantity of salt used.

How much salt is the minimum amount necessary for most people?

The most frequent estimate of the minimum daily adult requirement is 200 mg of sodium (0.5 grams of salt). However, most American consumers today eat from 3,900–4,700 mg (10 to 12 grams of salt). In 1977, the Senate Select Committee on Nutrition and Human Needs recommended a goal of five grams of salt a day to be added to raw foods as they are prepared commercially or at home including salt added at the table. This would be in addition to the three grams or so which already occur naturally in foods. It would bring the total salt recommendation by this Committee to eight grams daily, or a reduction of 20 percent of the salt from a diet containing ten grams. But recommendations of committees, especially political committees, are not always the best science!

A diet consisting of only 200 mg of sodium would be unpalatable to most people. However, a 20 percent reduction in salt intake might be a reasonable goal for many people. However, it is unreasonable to establish a single goal for all Americans because of the variations in salt requirements, tolerances, health, and nutritional status among different people.

The person who is overweight, at risk for high blood pressure, or subject to other health problems has a lower tolerance for salt than the rest of the population and should eat less salt. That does not necessarily mean that everyone should eat less salt. In the normal body, salt is not stored. Excess salt is released through sweat, feces, and urine (primarily).

Does everyone's blood pressure go up when salt is eaten?

No. That is one of the mysteries of the relationship of salt to high blood pressure. While the relationship has been under study for over 60 years, it is still not generally accepted that salt (sodium, specifically) causes high blood pressure, or hypertension.

The blood pressure of people in normally good health does not increase, even when they are fed amounts of sodium far above those usually consumed by Americans. However, the blood pressure of many unmedicated patients with hypertension will go down when the sodium in their diets is restricted (below a gram daily). And it will increase again when substantial amounts of sodium are returned to the diet.

Does everyone with high blood pressure eat a lot of salt?

Not everyone. Many, but not all, studies of various ethnic populations have indicated a positive correlation between the estimated average salt consumption and the incidence of high blood pressure. However, these studies are epidemiological, and often leave unaccounted other possible causes of hypertension, such as genetic predisposition, obesity, general nutritional status, and potassium intake. It is also very difficult to study the differences among individuals within the various cultures.

Is anyone ever salt deficient?

Yes, but rarely. Salt is essential to many of the physiological activities in man and all mammals. We would indeed be unhealthy, as well as unhappy, if we were to become salt deficient. In fact, we would be subject to headaches, weakness, dizziness, lack of concentration, poor memory, and poor appetite.

Why do you recommend that dietary salt be restricted?

Since sodium is known to play a major role in the physiological regulation of body fluids, it is reasonable to assume that it is capable of *influencing* blood pressure, whether or not it actually *causes* hypertension. For this reason, we advise everyone, and particularly those who are otherwise at risk for high blood pressure, to limit dietary salt. There may be no need to be drastic about it, but it may be useful to your future health to cut down (not eliminate) the amount of salty foods eaten and not to sprinkle salt on food at the table. However, salt must not be considered a total "badditive." It is an essential part of the human diet.

THE SALT OF THE EARTH

For various health reasons, people are placed on salt-free or low sodium diets. Sometimes this is recommended for people whose ankles swell, sometimes for stroke patients, and also for those with high blood pressure. Although these conditions are primarily medical problems, nutrition may play a role. Please note the use of the word *may*. Strokes are usually associated with an increase in blood pressure and a type of hardening of the arteries similar to that found in coronary heart disease. High blood pressure is frequently lowered by decreasing drastically the sodium content of the diet. This is done largely by restricting the use of salt, both in cooking and at the table. A moderate reduction in weight usually results in a decrease in an elevated blood pressure.

If you need to lower your salt intake, there are a few simple things you can do to begin to shift toward this new mode of eating. First of all, give your salt shakers away, both the one on the table and the one in the kitchen. Next, eat less of those foods which are prepared with added salt—for example, ham and potato chips. Depending on how low your diet should be in sodium, you may have to restrict milk and its products or use a low sodium milk preparation. Finally, be careful you are not getting substantial amounts of sodium in toothpaste or mouth washes. Ask your dentist or pharmacist to recommend low sodium products. Ask your doctor to get the American Heart Association booklets on sodium (or salt) restriction. There are three: for strict, moderate, and mild restriction. The foods to use and to avoid are very well outlined, and sample menus are given.

As if heart disease were not enough of a problem in menu planning, some people have a second health problem such as diabetes, which also must be considered in dietary management.

GENERAL DIET FOR HEART DISEASE AND DIABETES

One reader writes, "My mother has heart disease and diabetes which is controlled by oral medication. She thinks there is not a great deal of palatable food she can eat and feel good on. I contend there is. She eats a lot of food that doesn't add up to a good diet. Can you offer any suggestions?"

Depending on the type of heart disease and the severity of the diabetes, your mother can certainly have a wide variety of foods and a good diet. If the diabetes is well controlled by an oral preparation, it cannot be too severe. A diet moderately restricted in calories, carbohydrates, cholesterol, and salt should do it. Here is a specific, typical menu:

Breakfast	Fruit or juice
	Cereal with skim milk
	Toast (1 or 2 slices) with butter or margarine and no jam
	Coffee or tea
Lunch	Sandwich of
	Sliced chicken
	Lettuce
	Butter, margarine or mayonnaise
	Bread, 2 slices
	Banana
	Milk, tea, or coffee
Mid-afternoon	Fruit juice drink (½ soda water, ½ orange juice)
	2 graham crackers
Evening meal	Lean roast beef (no gravy)
	Parsley new potatoes
	Broccoli and lemon sauce
	Garden salad with French dressing
	Baked apple
	Bread and butter or margarine
	Tea or coffee (no sugar)
Bedtime	Glass of milk
	Cheese and crackers

The American Dietetic Association, 430 N. Michigan Ave., Chicago, IL 60611 has various meal planning aids available for people with diabetes. "Exchange Lists for Meal Planning" is one booklet available from this group, as are other useful pamphlets.

SEMANTICS AND POLICY

To us the modern fuss over diet and heart disease is largely a question of semantics, of not reading carefully the reports and recommendations of organizations such as the American Heart Association, the American Council on Science and Health, and various federal agencies, and of those in the media responsible for writing headlines and captions of news pieces.

A former colleague at Harvard, Dr. Mark Hegsted, recently Director of USDA's Human Nutrition Center, was quoted as saying: "Food is for nourishment and enjoyment. It was in this spirit that we presented the Dietary Guidelines—not as a panacea, a prescription, or a nutritional insurance policy." That statement is not very different from the following that appears in the recent report of the Food and Nutrition Board: "Sound nutrition is not a panacea. Good food that provides appropriate proportions of nutrients should not be regarded as a poison, a medicine, or a talisman. It should be eaten and enjoyed."

And for years and years, we at Harvard and at every other academic nutrition center, have taught that food is necessary for reasons of both physiology (to nourish) and psychology (to enjoy, among others). One of our "theme songs" has long been that eating is one of the pleasures of life. Also, that *variety* in foods consumed (variety among and within the Basic Four Food Groups) and *moderation* in amounts consumed are the keys to better nutrition.

Over the years, researchers have emphasized the multi-contributory nature of heart disease—heredity, blood pressure, smoking, level and type of cholesterol in the blood, obesity, physical activity, diabetes, and possibly stress. The American Heart Association refers to these contributing factors as "risk factors." The more of these risk factors one has, the greater the risk of heart disease. If you have none, the risk is slight. Many of these risk factors are influenced by obesity, even mild obesity. Thus, reduction in body weight to the range of Desirable Weight will usually result in a decrease in blood pressure, in blood cholesterol, and in the intensity of diabetes. Reduction of weight is best obtained by a combination of *consuming fewer calories* (from both food and drink) and *expending more* (physical activity). The latter also improves circulation and relieves stress.

The American Heart Association suggests that if you have some or all of the risk factors for heart disease, changes in your diet (and other changes in lifestyle) are important, and most researchers agree. The American Council on Science and Health suggests that "individual assessment and therapy based on an analysis of all suspected risk factors . . . multiple risk interpretations for the individual patient are superior to a campaign designed (only) to modify the American Diet." This statement is quite similar to one from the Food and Nutrition Board's recent report: "The Board considers it scientifically unsound to make single, all-inclusive recommendations to the public regarding intakes of various nutrients to decrease heart disease except to . . . adjust dietary energy intake and energy expenditure so as to maintain appropriate weight for height."

The completely healthy individual is one who does not have any of the risk factors and for whom manipulation of the diet—less saturated fat and less cholesterol—is therefore not necessary.

Dr. J. Michael McGinnis, Deputy Assistant Secretary for Health, said in a public statement, "The weight of existing evidence continues to suggest that for the U.S. population, as a whole, reduction in intake of total fat, saturated fat, and cholesterol would be sensible." We disagree and think this is an example of misplaced emphasis and more confusion for the public (and the health professionals). We would say, "The weight of existing evidence continues to suggest that for the U.S. population, as a whole, reduction in total *calories* and increase in *calorie* expenditure would be sensible."

So, what is the bottom line? It is that if you are a healthy American with none of the risk factors, consider yourself lucky. There is no evidence that reducing your intake of total fat, saturated fat, cholesterol, and salt, or increasing your intake of polyunsaturated fat is necessary. However, if you have some of the risk factors known to relate to diet—obesity, an elevated blood pressure, an elevated cholesterol level—then some dietary changes *may* be helpful, and the thoughtful, prudent individual should certainly make them.

And what are they? 1) Cut down on total caloric intake, which for most of us means less meat, less cheese and whole milk products, and less alcoholic beverages; 2) increase physical activity so you will use more energy. The combination of these two suggestions will result in weight loss and, usually, in a lowering of blood pressure and blood cholesterol; 3) if blood cholesterol is not decreased by this weight loss, then a decrease in saturated fats replaced by an increase in polyunsaturated fats, and a decrease in dietary cholesterol (fewer egg yolks, etc.) are in order; 4) if the weight loss does not result in a satisfactory decrease in blood pressure, then dietary salt should be reduced.

This all seems rather uncomplicated, so why all the confusion? Could it be that some politicians are interested in deliberately misinterpreting various reports in the hope of a little added publicity, or are they just misinformed?

And here's a tip for those of you who live where the snow falls deep and the snow removal equipment's efficiency may depend upon unsnarling a city's problems.

DIET SURVIVAL

When the Farmer's Almanac predicts heavy snow this winter, don't add to the problems by being an emergency yourself. Diabetics in particular, but actually anyone with definite and exacting dietary needs should always "be prepared." In an issue of its newsletter, the Greater Boston Diabetes Society printed some very important precautionary measures to be followed by diabetics. Avoid trouble by making plans. Disaster survival may depend on them.

1. Keep to your diet and insulin schedule as closely as possible. Give prompt attention to injuries. Keep warm and dry if at all possible.
2. Have a good supply of insulin on hand as well as extra needles and syringes. Be sure your sterilizing equipment is in proper order.
3. Keep on hand at least a 3-day supply of food for your diet. These foods should be stored easily, not require refrigeration, be safe from contamination, and be consumable without additional preparation. The following items fit these criteria: Canned meat or fish, Cheese in jars or carefully sealed packages, Canned vegetables and vegetable juices, Canned fruits and fruit juices, Evaporated milk, Packaged cereals, Canned soups, Salt, pepper, vinegar, and Mayonnaise or salad dressings. All bulk or packaged materials which have been in contact with flood water, silt, or other filth should be destroyed. Bottled foods with screw tops become contaminated if submerged. Frozen foods that have been thawed are not always safe.
4. Another very important point: anyone starting off on a trip during winter weather or on heavily traveled freeways should carry a box lunch in case of traffic tie-ups interfering with getting food on time.
5. Be sure you have your diabetic identification card with you at all times.
6. As far as utensils are concerned, a can opener is pretty important. And so is soap. You might also include: paper plates, cups, spoons, aluminum foil, matches, pans, and canned heat or a camp stove.

Remember, be ready to take care of yourself. Don't expect others to do it. They will be busy enough without adding you to their problems.

Another problem relating to carbohydrates is the rather uncommon condition known as hypoglycemia.

A WORD ON HYPOGLYCEMIA

Hypoglycemia means low blood sugar. Weakness, dizziness, and even fainting are common symptoms, and they usually occur one or two hours after meals, particularly after a skimpy breakfast. One who is really troubled with low blood sugar, and very few people are, may avoid the condition by increasing the amount of protein and fat in the diet and decreasing the sugar. As part of the treatment it is desirable to eat a substantial breakfast which is generous in protein and fat. This tends to avoid unusual fluctuation in the level of sugar in the blood, particularly the marked decreases that sometimes occur in midmorning. Food intake for the rest of the day should be divided into four or five small meals every three hours or so rather than just twice a day at noon and evening. At these times one should eat a regular, varied diet of foods providing protein, fat, and carbohydrate. In summary, protein and fat are actually increased moderately for the prevention and treatment of hypoglycemia, particularly at breakfast, and one consumes a number of small meals every day rather than the customary three. The purpose of all this is to avoid unusual fluctuation in the level of sugar in the blood and the accompanying weakness and dizziness.

Some other individuals, either because of physical abnormalities or nervous tension, will be more comfortable when they eat a bland diet.

AVOIDING IRRITATION

We receive many questions regarding diets for those people who are troubled by cramps, diarrhea, colitis, and "spastic colon." Actually, there are several very different causes for the inflammation called colitis. And "spastic colon" may result in diarrhea, constipation, or both of these conditions. Cramps and diarrhea may be caused by a variety of factors such as careless food and bowel habits, acute infection, serious disease, or even tension. Since so many different causes may result in similar symptoms, only a doctor can diagnose and prescribe exactly what is appropriate treatment for a specific individual.

However, a well-balanced diet, good nutrition, and the right weight are as necessary for persons with intestinal difficulties as for everyone else. Therefore, everyone who omits first this food and then that food because they may be "irritating" soon cuts out essential nutrients, too. The original problem is not cleared up, and becomes aggravated by poor nutrition. People who treat themselves on the basis of vague ideas about what is "bad" may suffer more from what they do *not* eat than from what they eat.

The experts are very careful not to eliminate too much. Many foods have been termed "binding" or "laxative" or "gas producers," but there is very little proof of the effect of individual foods on the intestine.

In recent years, diets high in fiber have been recommended for most people, even those with an irritable bowel and spastic colon. True, the typical American diet is low in fiber, but it is easy to increase the fiber content. Whole grain breads, bran-containing cereals, and vegetables and fruits are good sources of fiber, particularly those fruits that have edible skins such as plums and grapes.

It is thought by some that it is beneficial to restrict alcohol and coffee, as well as spicy and pickled foods. Certainly, with an "irritable colon," it is sensible for any individual to avoid any particular food which is found to be distressing. On the whole, however, worry about the effect of this or that food may be more harmful than the food itself, and cutting out many foods is definitely unwise. To concentrate on what and how to eat may be more beneficial than to try to figure out what not to eat.

Do see your doctor. Do establish good bowel habits and drink plenty of water. Do be sure your diet is well balanced and contains the number of calories that is right for you. Do eat meals regularly, and chew food thoroughly. Do exercise regularly. In other words, worry less, relax more, and stick with the Basic Four Food Groups.

Next come some thoughts on diet for gastritis sufferers.

RIGHT IN THE STOMACH

We want to emphasize one point, first of all, for all of you who complain of stomach problems. That point is simply this: see your doctor! A diet we might recommend for one person or one stomach ailment may not be right for you or for a member of your family. No one can prescribe for heartburn or gastritis or other stomach symptoms without knowing what is producing them. Only a physician who understands a patient and the cause of his trouble can give specific advice.

But we can explain certain general principles that are basic, and that may be helpful. We can also emphasize this: as much harm may be done by individuals who make their own diagnosis and their own diets as by any underlying disturbance. Some people think they should not eat tomatoes, oranges, or juices because they are "acid." Others believe meats or vegetables are bad for heartburn or gastritis. Actually, cutting out these foods just makes matters worse because the body is seriously depleted of necessary nutrients.

Other popular restrictions are equally senseless. There is very little experimental evidence to justify many of the commonly accepted ideas of what is good or bad, digestible or indigestible.

"Acidity" is another source of confusion. Hydrochloric acid is found in all normal stomachs and is required for digestion of food. No "acid" foods are as acid as this hydrochloric acid. However, gastric discomfort may be reduced if the normal stomach acid can be decreased or neutralized. To some extent, fats and proteins help to do this. However, relief is often best obtained through eating frequent small meals.

When "bland" diets are prescribed for gastric distress, the chemically irritating foods which are usually omitted are spices, coffee, alcohol, and the extractives in meat, soups, and gravies. Finally, foods which are thermally irritating are those which are very hot or ice cold. But there is little good evidence to support any of these eliminations. Much of this is psychological—but if it works, that's fine.

However, what is included is as important as what is excluded. The day's meals must include a good variety of all the Basic Four foods, and a correct number of calories. Nutrition needs to be maintained, and weight should be watched. Both over-nutrition and under-nutrition may create extra problems in any stomach condition. Proper eating habits are also a key part of the picture. Food should be well chewed, and meals should be regular and relaxed.

This is the basic pattern. Your doctor can help you fit it to your special requirements. Your doctor is also your adviser if you are having gallbladder problems.

THE GALL OF IT ALL

Wouldn't it be great if one could make the pain of gallstones disappear simply by changing to a different diet? Unfortunately, if one really has gallstones causing persistent pain, surgical treatment is usually the order of the day. People who occasionally have a collicky pain related to their gallbladder may get relief by eating smaller, more frequent meals. If it has been clearly shown that a meal rich in fats sets off an individual's gallbladder attack, fat restriction may be useful. However, for most gallbladder trouble, a well-balanced diet consumed in 5 or 6 small meals each day is the best solution.

As an interesting aside, it appears that in a very few individuals more pyridoxine and magnesium may be of value in lessening the formation of kidney and bladder stones. As far as is known, the vast majority of the population gets enough pyridoxine and magnesium (as well as other vitamins and minerals) from a well-balanced diet. Undoubtedly, there are some few individuals who, for unknown reasons, have an unusually high requirement for pyridoxine and magnesium. In such cases, it is necessary to give these nutrients as medications under a physician's prescription. Such a cause of stones clearly is the unusual exception, but is presented here simply as a matter of interest.

A BOUT WITH GOUT

If you are among those suffering from gout, there is little comfort to be derived from the knowledge that Benjamin Franklin also endured this problem. It would be far more comforting to think that you simply needed to change your style of eating to remove yourself from the roster of those with gout. You probably already know that the level of uric acid in the blood increases in an attack of gout.

Some years ago it was thought that foods high in substances called purines should be avoided by those who had gout. Such foods were meats, particularly glandular meats including liver or kidney. However, treatment of gout by means of a drug known as colchicine or another drug called Benemid®, is reasonably effective, much more so than diet. The low purine diet for gout is pretty much out of style because of its ineffectiveness. Gout is a very painful disease, though not serious. It should be treated by your physician.

Let's switch now to another health problem where diet may be important.

RASH ACTIONS

Some of your best friends have it—allergy, that is. Probably lots of your friends talk about it and discuss their interesting allergies. But not many really understand the allergy and its treatment. Yet a little knowledge can dispel many mistaken ideas, and life becomes easier for those who have allergies.

What is allergy? It's an unusual reaction to something which ordinarily is harmless. The cause of the reaction is a protein substance known as an allergen.

It can be something in the air that is breathed or in the food that is eaten. Allergic reactions can even be caused just by being in contact with an offending substance, or occasionally by sunlight or extremes of heat or cold. Allergy not only has many causes; it also has many effects. People with an allergy may develop hay fever or asthma, or symptoms such as rashes and skin problems, headaches, nausea, or diarrhea.

There are other differences which complicate this condition. In some persons the reaction to an allergen is immediate; in others it may be delayed a day or so. Also, the severity may be influenced by such factors as worry or unusual strain.

It is a big challenge, therefore, to discover just what is the source of the trouble. Detection requires expert skill and guidance. Foods most often found to be bothersome are milk, eggs, and grains. Other foods frequently involved are nuts, seeds, beef, pork, chocolate, tomatoes, and seafood.

In every case there is great individual variation. For instance, the amount that is hazardous may be tiny or large. Or a person who cannot drink ordinary bottled cow's milk may do very well on evaporated milk or on goat's milk.

Hidden allergens often create difficulty. Those who are allergic must learn to be good detectives, to look beneath the surfaces, and to read package contents carefully. Otherwise, there is no way of knowing what is concealed in bread or cake, batter or sauce.

Meal planning is strictly an individual matter. However, no matter what has to be eliminated, it is absolutely necessary to include all the basic nutritional essentials that everyone requires.

3

TIPS ON GOOD EATING FOR A LIFETIME

"Family plan" has long been a standard travel plan widely used by today's flying families. Now it is time to try this approach on menus, too. In the matter of food, a family plan can mean better fare for all. True, each age has certain special demands, but generally speaking, the whole family shares the same food needs.

What is more, early eating habits are lasting habits. A good start can be the beginning of better eating and better health for children and for their family, too. Good nutrition for all ages begins with ordinary food prepared and eaten in a pleasant atmosphere.

A healthful master plan provides the Basic Four: fruits and vegetables (including citrus fruit daily and dark green, leafy or yellow vegetables); whole grain or enriched bread and cereals; milk and other dairy products; and meat, fish, or poultry. Amounts have to be varied to meet the needs of various ages, but these foods are necessary every day from childhood to old age.

A healthful master plan provides three wholesome meals as the ordinary daily pattern. It means a sit-down breakfast for everyone, a nourishing lunch, and a well-balanced dinner. For some individuals this may be varied to include more frequent, but smaller meals or nourishing snacks.

Finally, wise planning adjusts portion sizes. Then each person is encouraged to maintain his own best weight, an idea just as important to the very young and the very old as it is to the weight-conscious teenager.

Within the basic blueprint, there can be minor modifications for different family members. Yet a mashed food here, a change in quantity there, does not alter the overall pattern.

63

For instance, allowance must be made for the appetite lull of the pre-schooler. The toddler may tire of food and want very little. However, even though his servings are small, he can learn to establish good nutrition habits if he joins the family table and if the family food is well planned. A little one is well on his way to growing up when he copies the other members of his family who are eating a variety of wholesome foods in normal amounts.

School brings renewed appetite. Habits of good eating are very important in this time of great activity, childhood diseases, and frequent colds.

During adolescence, food patterns frequently are put to a big test, particularly by girls. Children who grow rapidly during the teens must have foods that build strong bones and muscles. Furthermore, future mothers need to be storing nutrients for the coming years. The seemingly insatiable appetite of the teenage boy usually prompts him to eat a reasonable amount of food, but fads and the desire to be "model-thin" frequently lead the adolescent girl into poor nutrition habits if she has not formed strong habits of eating well. Chances are that pre-teens and teenagers will get the necessary nutrients if they have formed the habit of eating regularly and if they see the rest of the family eating sensibly.

The family plan benefits parents, too. They need nourishing foods that repair and maintain body tissues during the years of stress and strain, of waking early and working late.

And Grandma and Grandpa? Often they are tempted to stint, sometimes to stuff. A pattern of good habits will help them tremendously to eat wisely in these sometimes difficult years.

A good food plan can fill the bill for the whole family and help each member develop and enjoy healthful habits for a lifetime of good eating.

On the surface, good nutrition sounds like a realistic expectation for anyone who has at least a minimum income and an ordinary endowment of common sense. It is obvious that good nutrition is very possible to achieve and clearly bears rewards for anyone who eats the appropriate amounts of each of the nutrients. However, the various stages of life each carry certain elements that may complicate eating practices.

BREAST-FEEDING

One of the most important decisions you (and your husband) will make before your baby is born is whether to breast-feed or bottle-feed your newborn. There are pluses and minuses on both sides of the breast-feeding question for parents in the United States and other developed nations, and there is no definitive evidence that one answer or the other is correct for all people. Thus, the decision needs to be considered on an individual basis by each family along with their doctor.

In the 1940s, approximately 65 percent of all babies born in the United States were breast-fed, but that number had dropped to only 15 percent in 1972. This situation has undergone an important reversal in the past few years as a result of considerable publicity about breast-feeding. The LaLeche League is the organization which has dedicated its efforts intensively toward encouraging breast-feeding and aiding new mothers in their efforts to nurse their infants.

Success in breast-feeding is not related to breast size and seldom is related to nipple shape. Dr. Mary Ellen Avery, Physician-in-Chief of the Children's Hospital Medical Center in Boston, and Dr. Ilene R. S. Sosenko at Harvard Medical School feel that women who want to breast-feed and are taught the proper method have a 95 percent chance of success in nursing their infants. The nursing infant stimulates the nerve endings in the nipples, which stimulates the brain to produce two hormones—prolactin, which stimulates the breast to produce milk, and oxytocin, which causes the ejection of milk to the nipple. As long as the breast is stimulated by the nursing baby, it will produce milk, and the more it is stimulated, the more milk it will produce.

The Committee on Nutrition of the American Academy of Pediatrics and the Nutrition Committee of the Canadian Pediatric Society have endorsed breast milk as providing the newborn infant better nutrition with more immunologic factors than formulas or cow's milk. Information from the study of these two committees, plus the comments of Drs. Avery and Sosenko follow:

1. Lipids (fats) are absorbed better by the newborn from breast milk than from cow's milk or infant formulas, but newer formulas closely resemble breast milk in their fat composition.
2. Iron from human milk is absorbed better than that from cow's milk (which is lower in lactoferrin, an iron-binding protein) and is plentiful enough for breast feeding to be the sole source of iron until the birth weight is tripled. However, the iron in formulas also can be absorbed well as a consequence of a special heat treatment.
3. Cholesterol content is higher in breast milk than in vegetable oil formulas and may have significance in later life, either in relation to bile salt synthesis or nerve tissue or by inducing enzymes to improve cholesterol metabolism. This area is in need of additional research before conclusions can be drawn.
4. Proteins from human milk are more digestible and more attuned to infant needs than are the proteins in cow's milk. However, some milk-based formulas have been modified so that the proteins resemble those in human milk rather closely.
5. In human milk, the sodium and other mineral contents are lower, which may be better suited to the infant's needs than is true for cow's milk, but milk-based formulas have been modified now to match human milk rather closely.

There are definite immunological benefits to breast milk, for it provides active leukocytes, with antibodies to fight off intestinal infections, and with immunoglobulins to ward off respiratory and other infections; its lactoferrin inhibits some of the intestinal infections. However, new babies are born with their own set of immunities, which should suffice to protect them for a few months no matter which milk is being fed.

With these facts in mind, consider now some practical matters that might influence your decision-making. With breast-feeding, you never have to worry about bottles you've forgotten to wash. You also don't have to remember to buy formula. Breast-feeding can also be cheaper than bottle-feeding. You will need to eat a good diet in slightly larger quantities than you would eat in your pre-pregnancy days, but such costs can be controlled with good menu planning and marketing.

Breast-feeding does require that you be available for baby's meals. With bottle-feeding, someone else can enjoy the baby's feeding time while you rest. Breast-feeding will not allow you to know exactly how much nourishment your baby is getting, but you can be sure the food is adequate if normal weight gain is occurring. There is little likelihood that the baby will be overfed because most of the milk is expressed during the first three to six minutes of nursing time.

So either breast or bottle-feeding can be done—the choice belongs to you. By either method, you can be a good parent. Regardless of the method of feeding, be sure to cuddle your infant close to you—and invite the new father to cuddle close, too!

BABY FOODS

Commercial baby foods and home-prepared baby foods are equally acceptable for your infant—as long as proper nutritional and safety precautions are taken. The commercial baby foods have the advantage of being able to process the fruits and vegetables at their peak of freshness and nutritional value, a situation which sometimes cannot be duplicated at home. Home prepared foods have the advantage of being able to be prepared and fed without having to undergo the canning process.

Parents are concerned about some aspects of commercially prepared baby foods, which has led to some changes in their preparation in the last few years. The amount of salt added to baby foods has been reduced in response to consumer concern, and monosodium glutamate (MSG) has been eliminated from baby foods. In fact, some baby foods do not have any salt added to them either. Sugar content of commercial baby foods also is being shifted downward.

If the water content of commercial baby foods is of concern to you, consider that all foods contain a large amount of water. An apple, for example, is about 90 percent water. Labeling regulations require the listing of ingredients in descending order, a requirement which places water near the first on the list. Water needs to be included in various baby foods at comparatively high levels in order to give them the appropriate consistency for easy swallowing.

Some people have questioned the use of modified food starches in baby food, complaining that they are just "fillers". On the contrary, modified food starches, derived from corn or tapioca starch, are excellent sources of carbohydrates—an essential part of a baby's diet. In addition, unmodified starches break down in storage, whereas modified starches have good shelf-life. Modified starches serve to stabilize the food to which they are added so that separation is prevented, and the food consistency is not only kept uniform, but is improved so that the food is appetizing and easy to swallow. The safety of modified starches has been established unequivocally by the Food and Drug Administration and the National Academy of Sciences after thorough examination and evaluation. Using modified starches to increase palatability (at levels between 4 and 6 percent) is an advantage that commercial baby foods have over those prepared in the home.

A word of caution about the feeding of baby food is appropriate here. Never feed a baby directly from the jar of baby food unless all the food will be eaten at one meal. Returning the spoon again and again to the jar after it has been in the mouth returns saliva to the food. While the leftover food is being stored, the saliva begins to contaminate the food in the jar with increased microbiological levels and also breaks down the starch. To help avoid such contamination, pour the desired amount of food from the jar into another container for feeding and promptly refrigerate the covered remainder of the container.

If you prepare all of your baby's food at home, you'll have other safety precautions to worry about also. Home preparation demands a lot of time and trouble, and you might prefer to spend that time doing other things with your baby, but that is your own decision. However, when introducing a new food to a baby, where only a teaspoon or less will be used, it does seem a bit impractical to go through all the fuss and bother of starting from scratch.

As your baby gets a little older, when sterilization is no longer necessary (although you would be exercising similar principles of sanitation, anyway), and it's time to switch from baby food to "table food," you might want to use your blender. You'll find the junior foods which are available commercially are very little different from what your baby has already been eating. With the aid of a blender, you'll be able to serve many of the foods from your table in lieu of buying junior foods.

Another word of caution is to be sure to avoid forcing your baby to eat every morsel you have prepared. Feed only the amount your baby seems to want. That food can suitably be either your home-prepared or commercially prepared baby and junior foods. Remember that millions of babies have been raised very successfully by both methods.

Can babies be well nourished from commercial baby foods?

Certainly. It is estimated that, since baby foods were introduced more than 40 years ago, at least 150 million American infants have received nutritionally adequate diets from their use. There is no dispute among recognized authorities that commercial baby foods do provide adequate nutrition for infants. One advantage to commercial baby foods is that a mother knows exactly what she is getting, because the Recommended Dietary Allowances (RDA) are listed on the labels.

Isn't it true that mothers who make their own baby foods are giving their infants more nutritious food?

No. Baby food companies use top-quality ingredients, processed when they are at their maximum nutritional value. In contrast, when a mother buys "fresh" foods at the store, they may be days old before she gets them home, and they may have lost some of their nutritive quality. In addition, it is impossible to get the variety of fruits and vegetables to meet the nutritional needs of the baby on a year-round basis. They simply are not available in the stores. So the truth is that a mother cannot duplicate the efforts of the baby food companies in this respect. Baby foods were first put on the market to fill a great need—the need for a convenient and easy way to provide baby with the variety of foods doctors were prescribing. In fact, they have liberated mothers from a time-consuming job, and generations of satisfied mothers and healthy children can attest to their value.

FOOD HABITS

We are all aware of the extensive evidence gathered over the years clearly indicating the need for good nutrition. Time and again it has been demonstrated that enough (but not too much) of the right food is necessary for the best possible growth and well-being. Yet people still do not eat well even here in the United States where there is enough food for everyone. Far too many do not eat what they need for optimum health and appearance.

Teenage boys and girls put their trust in snacks. They may skip meals and skimp on the foods that are needed for vigor and accomplishment, for good looks and a good physique.

Adults, too, eat too little at one meal, too much at another. Some are skinny; some are weak and weary; and many are simply too fat.

Why are these foolish practices so common? The answer does not lie simply in the availability of food. More and more, it has been recognized that eating is not merely a matter of meals and menus. Many factors enter into the picture. Careful and extensive studies from several states have shown that we need to understand the reasons for poor nutrition habits if the situation is to be improved. For instance, a person's attitude toward food is influenced by the way he was fed in infancy and childhood. Unpleasant experiences associated with eating leave their mark on eating habits. Often tense or miserable individuals seek relief from tensions and anxieties through the satisfaction food provides them; they eat and eat, and finally become the people who are forever trying unsuccessfully to lose weight. Other unhappy individuals meet their emotional needs by refusing to eat. Perhaps they are trying to attract attention, or they may be trying in a very subtle way to punish another person. Such behavior can be seen quite transparently in some children's performances at the family dinner table.

Sometimes young people "follow the leader" and pick up patterns that are supposed to bring popularity with the gang. Frequently, misguided young persons think they have no time for breakfast or lunch. In other cases, idleness leads to poor habits. In Iowa it was found that young girls ate better in the winter when they had a regular routine than in the summer when they had plenty of free time.

These are but a few of the possible factors influencing your food habits. Actually, there are multiple factors such as religion, food myths, experience, economics, education, health, work and play habits, profits, competition, and many others that influence us to eat the foods we habitually choose.

Many practical matters also affect food habits, for example, processing, transportation, and storage facilities for food. These represent enormous problems in feeding populations locally or world-wide.

Man's feelings and attitudes about food are deeply rooted in his nature and culture. As processing techniques developed, it was found that refined food such as white flour rather than dark whole wheat flour, polished rice rather than unpolished, and white sugar rather than brown had better keeping qualities. In addition to better keeping qualities, these items were preferred by those of the upper social classes, and hence a status symbol was attached to them. As people struggled to move up the social ladder, they reached out to buy these overt symbols of success as one means of helping the rest of the world note their achievement. There was also the subtle implication that the whiteness of these refined foods indicated a higher degree of purity and safety.

Good food habits to most of us generally mean the habits with which we are familiar, and which we practice—but this does not necessarily mean these habits are good from the viewpoint of health. Custom is an unwritten law of life, and it is difficult to change.

Not only is food steeped in tradition, but social customs may determine to varying degrees what one eats and with whom. In some cultures, women and children may not eat with men. The men eat first, the children next, and the women last. Foods thought to be good for men are considered bad for women in some cultures. Where food is limited in quantity and quality, it is obvious who gets the best and the most. Remnants of those taboos exist today in most of our cities, although women's liberation activities may soon make the "men's dining room" and side entrances for women at some private clubs a memory of the past.

PRE-SCHOOL NUTRITION NEEDS MET (WITHOUT USE OF THREAT)

Many grandparents share a common concern as they watch their own children begin to raise the next generation. How easy it is to see the errors that are being made in feeding infants and pre-schoolers! From the comfortable distance of the second generation, the developing attitudes toward food and the instilling of food preferences come sharply into focus and it becomes easy to tell the parents, whose perception may be hampered by the closeness of their offspring, how you used to do it.

Sometimes it is a remarkable, if not alarming revelation to inventory what a child actually views as food he will eat. Some children drink milk, milk, and more milk, to the exclusion of virtually all other foods. Others may specialize in hamburgers with an occasional hot dog interspersed for variety. More adventurous, but still very limited young diners may broaden acceptance to fish sticks, hamburger, bacon, a cereal, and milk. Now these are all good foods, but they do not add up to a balanced diet by themselves. Fruits, vegetables, eggs, and a variety of cereals and meats are important additions at any age. These foods contain valuable nutrients, and they also do a great deal to add variety and pleasure to eating. Early introduction to a wide variety of foods makes eating more interesting throughout life and also avoids problems when one dines out. Who wants to be hostess to the person who thinks the world of food begins and ends with hamburgers and hot dogs? How many recipes are possible for a fancy dinner which has to feature bologna if one of your guests is to be made happy?

Yes, childhood clearly is the time to help people learn to enjoy food. Parents are shirking a responsibility and an opportunity when they content themselves with the idea that their children won't eat vegetables and many other foods. Teaching a child to eat properly and seeing that he receives a good, varied diet takes patience, understanding, and some knowledge combined with common sense. It is easy to give youngsters a bottle of milk and feel that good nutrition is taken care of. Unfortunately, milk is not a totally perfect food, although it is an excellent one. Milk, as the mainstay of the diet, lacks iron, vitamin C, and is low in calories and solids for a child more than 12 months old. Milk is an important part of a child's diet, but clearly is not a substitute for one or two spoonsful of vegetables, fruits, and other foods that, along with milk, form the basis of a good diet.

A child being weaned should sooner or later learn to taste and enjoy many different foods, and the sooner he does, the better his nutrition will be. Good eating habits can affect a whole life, but even the smartest infant isn't born with this knowledge. He doesn't know that bodies, like buildings, must have a sturdy foundation. He has to be taught, and this usually is done by his parents.

It is true that the learning period in child feeding may have its maddening moments. For a while, the very young infant may have some difficulty moving the first solid foods he eats to the back of his mouth where they can be swallowed easily. Instead, he may shove the food right back out of his mouth, not necessarily because he doesn't like it, but simply because he hasn't yet learned how to handle it. To the annoyance and consternation of the adult feeding him, the food may be returned from his mouth with a velocity never anticipated when he was given the spoonful. It is only natural for a busy parent to be tempted to put off the messy and time-consuming tasks of introducing new foods and helping children gradually learn to feed themselves.

However, a few smart approaches nearly always shorten and simplify the task. Often just by being calm a parent avoids tentative resistance to tasting a new food. Also, a wise parent introduces a new food when a child is hungry at the beginning of a meal and may be more willing and interested in trying something new. If he isn't interested in trying it, ignore the matter and offer it again some other time. Sometimes a new food will need to be offered several times before it begins to seem familiar and to appeal to the very young "gourmet."

There is a cheering reward for the mother who patiently strives to broaden a child's experiences with food. When a baby is taught good food habits early, he rapidly outgrows his need for special planning and preparation to meet his specific needs. In a short time he is ready to eat what is served to the whole family. Secondly, lack of appetite, listlessness, and picky attitudes toward food simply are not a problem. It is amazing how habits that are established early in life tend to be perpetuated throughout life. When these habits lead to good nutrition, food will never be a problem.

The fact that good nutrition is essential for optimum growth and development certainly should not be ignored. In some children the bad effects of hit-or-miss eating may not become apparent until some time later when the body is subjected to the added strain of the adolescent growth spurt, or childbearing, or old age.

There is no doubt about it: strength in all these years needs a foundation of good food in the first years. And in these first years, responsibility for a child's food and attitudes toward eating are clearly up to the parents!

Since children throughout the school years have a good many tests, let's turn the tables now and let you have the pleasure of taking a small quiz on nutrition.

CHILD NUTRITION QUIZ

What an infant is fed during just the first year is crucial for all the years that follow. Healthy minds and healthy bodies depend on eating healthful foods. So if you have anything to do with feeding youngsters, we hope you can pick the right answers in this quiz.

1. What determines how much a person will grow?
   a. Food is the important factor.
   b. Heredity is the important factor.

The answers are both correct. The growth limits which a person can reach are set by heredity long before birth. However, whether an individual will reach these limits is determined after birth by the food he eats. Why? Because food provides the building materials for bones, muscles, and body tissues. Only with enough of the right food at the right time can children grow and gain as they should.

2. Is mental development also influenced by food?
   a. It may not be affected by food.
   b. Food makes a big difference.

The answer is b. And there is no time to waste, because a person's brain reaches 70 per cent of its full size by the age of one, and it requires excellent nutrition for full development. Later on, poor nutrition may depress a child's IQ or slow up emotional development. Also, a child who does not have an adequate diet lacks the strength required for good mental performance.

3. If an infant is underfed at first and then well fed later on, what happens?
   a. He never makes up for the growing time he lost.
   b. He may recover completely.

Unfortunately, a is true. If a child has been seriously deprived of certain essential nutrients, especially protein and calories, it may not be possible for him to overcome this early handicap completely. Even though he may start growing quite rapidly if he finally receives all the nutrients he needs, he still is unlikely to attain his full potential height. Therefore, from the day of birth every child should be properly fed. If this has not been done, the situation should be remedied as promptly as possible.

4. Are commercial baby foods desirable?
   a. They are satisfactory, but not essential.
   b. They are preferable to home-prepared foods.

The first answer is correct. It is perfectly all right if a mother thinks commercial foods are too costly and prefers to use a food mill or strainer to make the family foods suitable for the baby. Or it is perfectly fine if she prefers to feed the commercial foods because they are convenient and easy to use and are less spicy than the rest of the family food.

What is most important is for the food to be well chosen and appealing. If babies learn early to eat and enjoy a wide variety of nutritious foods, they will have an excellent start toward good health. And when they reach adolescence and early adulthood they are less likely to develop emotional problems linked to food idiosyncrasies.

5. Are plump or fat infants healthier and better able to withstand childhood diseases than slightly lighter children?
   a. Yes, definitely true.
   b. No.

If you answered "b," you are in agreement with a growing number of pediatricians who feel that fatness in infants is to be avoided just as it is at all other ages. As for the concern with childhood diseases, good public health and well baby care plus good medical treatment and good, but not over-nutrition are all important.

6. Are vitamin supplements useful in feeding infants?
   a. No, adequate intake of milk assures an adequate supply of vitamins.
   b. Yes, infants may have too small an intake of food to provide adequate amounts of all of the vitamins even when they are "good eaters."

Again, the second answer is correct. Most pediatricians prescribe a multivitamin preparation for infants and young children to insure that they are getting the necessary amounts of vitamins. We think the preparation should also contain fluoride to promote strong teeth.

It is wise to take a good and impartial look at the way a child is eating, and this needs to be done frequently because children can change their habits and likes so often. Only by trying to view eating patterns of the family through the eyes of a stranger can you begin to appreciate the influences that are shaping the children.

WEIGHT (NOT WAIT) CONTROL

Children are often fed not wisely, but too well. Roundness may be pretty in pink-cheeked infants, but extra fat is not pretty at all in the chubby child, the husky pre-teen, the flabby teenager, or the obese adult. The plumpness that is sometimes considered pleasing in infants becomes unattractive and downright dangerous in everyone else, and may not even be healthy for the infant.

The time to act is early. An ounce of prevention in childhood eliminates pounds of misery later. Your child is lucky if you are teaching him good food habits while he is young.

However, if you are urging on him more food than he needs, you are contributing to fatness, not to health. The worst of it is that it gets harder and harder to break the habit of eating too much. Children should be taught early that there is a vital difference between good eating and over-eating.

What every youngster needs is a family that helps him follow a wise dietary regime. If the child's doctor thinks weight loss is indicated, then it is up to the family to help the overweight child get back to normal. This need not, and should not, include scolding and squabbling. Nothing at all is accomplished if the child is nagged, reproached, or deprived of too much. He becomes irritated and rebels against the rules altogether. He will follow a food plan far better if the diet is made as easy and painless as possible. This is a challenge for parents as well as for children. If the whole family follows a wise eating pattern, the child does better and everyone benefits.

If you want to help your children, there are many ways to cut corners and calories, too. Select snacks wisely. Encourage fresh fruit, celery, carrots, radishes, and pickles—all of them low in fat value and high in filling value.

There are other tricks. Reduce the size of portions. Cut down, rather than out. Remember, too, that slow eating can make food last longer. If a child is reminded to eat slowly, chances are that he will tend to eat more sparingly.

What else can you do to help your child reduce? Offer vinegar and lemon juice instead of mayonnaise and other salad dressings. Trim away meat fat so that it won't be a temptation. Substitute skim milk for whole; leave out butter pats, or slice them thinner. Try cutting creamy sauces, fried food, pie, cake, and pastry from the family menus. Finally, vary the foods as much as you can, and then dress them up! Pep up the servings with parsley or relish; top desserts with low calorie whips or a spot of jam. A diet is far easier when it is glamorized!

Last but not least, encourage exercise. Activity burns up stored fat and some of the calories in food. All too often overweight children are the ones who hate to move. They leave the gym and the swim to others; they like cheering, not playing. Yet they are the ones who most need physical activity.

Here, too, they can be helped by their families if everyone walks or exercises. With patience and planning, parents can make an overweight child happier now and healthier in the future. If all of the family joins in to get slim and stay slim, they will be happier and healthier, too.

Once children start school, the responsibility for good nutrition for the student is shared by the family and the school.

Tips for Teenagers

If you are a teenager or if you have a teenager in the family, you'll want to be aware of some of the problems teenagers face when trying to control their weight. A fat teenager is not necessarily a happy teenager, but instead may be subject to ridicule and discrimination from peers.

Even more important is the fact that the fat teenager is endangering future health. The development of atherosclerosis is accelerated, the metabolic system is overburdened, and psychological stress is heightened by excess weight. Even though dieting may be difficult during these years, many teenagers have done it successfully.

If you're a teenager, be cautious. Stop yourself from grabbing one of those fad diets that limits you to only a few foods. They may be eliminating some essential nutrients, too. Remember that you are still a growing person and need the right combinations of foods every day in order to function and grow optimally. Beware of tablets and candies that are a part of some diet plans.

Your best bet for planning a healthy reducing diet is to eat three meals a day, selecting a variety of foods from the Basic Four Food Groups and keeping the portions small, particularly for those foods that are high in energy such as meats and whole milk products. You may have learned about the Basic Four in school: 1) fruits and vegetables; 2) grains, such as bread and cereal; 3) milk and dairy products; and 4) meat, fish, or poultry. Choose a good diet and stick to it, serving yourself small portions which are perhaps half the size of those you served previously.

And eat slowly! Play a game with yourself and see how slowly you can eat one bite. It's a question of mind over matter. You possess the mind already; now make it work for you.

Some teenagers like to join a diet group for moral support. If this is not your idea of fun, try looking around you to see if anyone else you know could stand to lose a few pounds, also. When you find some fellow "plumpies," approach them and talk them into dieting with you. You can form your own diet group, make some new friends and have fun while slimming your way to better health.

You should include a self-styled exercise session—running around the block, stretching and bending, jumping rope, playing tag, tennis, dodge-ball or dancing. Exercise is important at all times, but especially when you are trying to lose weight. The weight is lost when more calories are burned up (during physical activity) than are taken in by the body from food or drink.

In general, you should not skip meals in order to lose weight, because that will just make you extra hungry when the next meal comes around, and you will want desperately to make up for the lost food by eating too much.

Breakfast is especially important. While you've been sleeping, your body has been growing and repairing, using the food you ate the day before. It needs refueling in the morning. Why should you torture yourself after a breakfastless morning by enduring the agony of a growling, empty stomach that constantly reminds you of how hungry you are and thus tempts you to snack on the wrong things—calorie-laden foods like candy or potato chips. Both of these can be included in your reducing diet, but in moderation.

Lunchtime is refueling time again, but refueling doesn't require a whole platter of food. Surprisingly little food is necessary for this meal. If school lunches seem to tempt you too strongly to overload your tray, then try brown-bagging your own lunch.

Get your mother's help, too. When she knows that you are serious about dieting, she will help you (or perhaps you can help her) with the grocery shopping, keeping in mind the caloric content of the various foods you select from each of the Basic Four Food Groups.

Snack times are the most dangerous times—while doing homework, watching TV, unwinding after a busy school day. If you must snack, remember that an apple contains only 80 calories, and a candy bar, depending on the size, may contain over 200.

Explore the delicious world of fresh fruits and vegetables—carrots, celery, and unsweetened juices. While candy, doughnuts, potato chips, cookies, pretzels, and soft drinks won't hurt you, they are loaded with calories and must be taken in small amounts only. If it's energy you are looking for, try orange juice after school. You might be surprised at how nicely that seems to wake you up, just as it does in the morning for breakfast.

Dinner can be dangerous, with its temptations to consume a huge meal in the evening to make up for your carefulness during the day. Here it is important to take small helpings of everything, even getting in the habit of using a small dinner plate. Remember that soon you will be sleeping and therefore burning up fewer calories than you did during the physically active day. Dinnertime is a good time to see how slowly you can eat. It also is a good time to replace the desire to eat too much with some stimulating conversation that will occupy your mind more than the food does.

If you are out with a date who is a non-dieter, concentrate on what your date would like to eat and do. Simply state that you are on a diet and immediately change the subject, while you order fresh fruit lemonade, unsweetened, and then sweeten it with a pack of the low-cal sweetener you always carry with you.

If you've been planning to diet, start now. No matter what day it is or what you are doing, you CAN make it work.

LOOKING OVER THE TEENS

There are good reasons for concern about the food habits of teenagers. First, nutritional demands in this period are at their maximum. The growth spurt preceding sexual maturation generally occurs in girls between ages 11 and 13 and in boys between ages 13 and 15. Bodies grow rapidly then. Indeed, in the ages 14 to 16, a girl's body requires more nutrients than at any other time in her life, with the exception of pregnancy and lactation. For a boy, the peak nutritional demands occur around ages 14 to 18.

Second, adolescents are generally casting off their habits of childhood and trying to establish their own identities. Part of this struggle may be the rejection of the diet advice they have been getting at home. As a result, too often teenagers are careless, skipping breakfast, going on fad diets, and filling up on snack foods, which by themselves do not provide good nutrition. This time of transition is also a period of emotional upheaval, a condition which often makes healthy eating difficult, although not impossible.

Third, teenagers are well-known for their susceptibility to fads—including fad diets. As we'll discuss below, some of these food fascinations can pose serious health problems.

Fourth, the habits formed as a teenager lay the groundwork for the entire adult eating pattern. It is important that, from the beginning, the expressions of individuality in the diet department place emphasis on nutritious, well-balanced meals.

It's never too early to think about good nutrition habits. We know, for instance, that our thousands of annual heart attack victims do not succumb because of what they ate in their 50s and 60s. Their susceptibility to this disease started many, many years before, and we feel that diet may have a great deal to do with that susceptibility. Some years ago, doctors performing autopsies on young American soldiers were startled to discover that many of them already had signs of atherosclerosis (fatty deposits causing narrowing) in their arteries, although the average age was only 22. The beginnings of this atherosclerosis probably began early in adolescence, or even earlier.

What are good healthy eating habits, both in the teen years and later? Skim or low-fat milk, more fish and chicken, and fewer egg yolks, as well as substituting polyunsaturated fats for saturated fats are all useful habits. Above all, fewer total calories, thus smaller portions are wise.

First, we must not forget that one out of every four mothers has her first child when she is less than 20 years old. So for a significant minority of teenage girls, the nutrition requirements involve more than just one person.

"Do as I say, not as I do" won't work when it comes to good food habits. Teenagers cannot do it alone. They need help, and this requires understanding and cooperation of parents and teachers. When teenagers are concerned about being fat or skinny, weak or weary, it is up to the adults to be available for advice. It is up to the leaders to set good examples and to practice what they preach. Too often mother sets the pattern, and daughter follows suit, in the no-breakfast routine. For the rest of the day, they cut down on meat, avoid bread and milk, and the vegetables and fruits may be few. What happens? They end up anemic.

Thousands and thousands of high school girls all over the land do not get enough iron. They lack zip. They are not alert for classes and dates. Iron-rich foods just cannot be ignored.

Boys skimp on lunch. Then at dinner, like so many of their fathers, they go light on fruits and vegetables, but heavy on pie and cake. Is that the kind of menu served at a training table? No! Athletes know that food makes a difference.

Watch the corner store near the high school before school starts in the morning. It is mobbed with youngsters grabbing a quick "breakfast" before classes—something quick like soft drinks and a candy bar. Nothing wrong with including either one occasionally as part of the day's intake, but they do not make a good substitute for breakfast, or any other meal. The calories are there, but there is a dearth of health-building nutrients. To be fit, adults as well as children must base their meals on the balance between the food groups. No one can cut nutritional corners consistently and come out on top.

Parents of teens and even pre-teens should aim to have their boys and girls receiving a well-balanced diet before the stage of the capricious appetite, the "herd" influence, the fascination with the bizarre are manifested in the teens. A youngster who has had sound training in good food habits does not persist in bad ones too long.

Furthermore, healthful, attractive meals can and should be served at home at regular times. When possible, the whole family should be expected to be there and to eat at least small portions of everything.

Good food habits must be a joint project for mothers and fathers and teenagers together. Are you parents helping your teenagers eat properly for strength now and health in the future? Are *you* setting good examples?

ACNE AND ADOLESCENCE

Acne is a comparatively common curse of adolescence, a problem of concern and confusion to many youngsters.

Is it true that chocolate is no longer regarded as a cause of acne?

For many years it has been well established that chocolate does not cause acne—nor does any other component of the diet that in the past has been associated commonly with acne. The actual cause, or causes, are very complex, and not all the answers are in yet. The condition is known to be influenced by hormone changes that occur in puberty, as well as by bacteria and other factors.

What are some of the other factors? Are any of them foods or chemicals found in foods?

Common factors associated with acne are certain cosmetics, particularly those that are oily or greasy and may plug up skin ducts. Humidity sometimes aggravates the condition, as do certain medications, such as steroids, iodide, and Dilantin.

If by "chemicals" in foods, you mean food additives, none has ever been shown to cause acne. However, certain "health food" products may aggravate the condition—kelp tablets, for instance, contain iodide which, as we have just mentioned, is often a factor. There no longer appears to be any relationship whatsoever between acne and commonly eaten foods.

I have read recently about a new vitamin A treatment for acne. Could you tell me more about it? Does it really work?

The treatment you have asked about is a synthetic form of vitamin A known as 13-cis-retinoic acid, a substance dermatologists have been familiar with for a number of years. The compound—and its potential value—is "new" only to the general public, after the news media featured a success story of its use in 14 severe and highly resistant cases. The report of its dramatic results was carried in the *New England Journal of Medicine*, but several more years of safety testing are needed before the product can be released for general use. Even then, it probably will be reserved for those who do not respond to other forms of treatment. 13-Cis-retinoic acid probably never will be used for women of childbearing age, because of its likelihood of causing birth defects.

Can't regular vitamin A supplements be used as treatment instead? Wouldn't they be safer?

This is one of the dangers of all the recent vitamin A publicity. Many persons do not understand that the form of vitamin A mentioned in the news story is far different from that found in ordinary vitamin A supplements. Doctors are concerned that sufferers will self-medicate with vitamin A "megadoses", a practice that could be extremely hazardous.

Vitamin A is a fat-soluble vitamin, meaning that excess amounts are not excreted from the body. Instead, the overload is stored in body fat, particularly that in the liver, and leads to possible liver damage and other serious side effects. **NEVER self-prescribe high doses of any vitamin or mineral supplement.**

SALUTING THE SCHOOL LUNCH

In November of 1981, the U.S. Department of Agriculture submitted to the President a revised version of their proposal for a reduction in the size of the school lunches. The current school lunch is required to supply approximately one-third of the daily nutritional requirements of a student 10 to 12 years of age. The new proposed reduction would require schools to serve a "tasting" portion of each of the five meal components (meat, milk, bread, fruit, and vegetables) rather than requiring children to take a full portion of each. An option would be to serve full-size portions of at least three components and "tasting portions" of the other items. Lunches would therefore offer fewer calories, fewer nutrients, and less total food, but would still provide approximately one-third of the recommended dietary allowances.

Critics of this proposal are worried that the new school lunch programs will be nutritionally inadequate. They fear that the reduced portion sizes will result in nutritional deficiencies and hungry, fatigued school children dragging through their afternoon classes. They also protest the increased flexibility of the new feeding program and are opposed to the idea of having "tasting portions" of several foods in place of larger servings.

Informed parents, however, should support the government's proposal for two primary reasons: almost 20 percent of school-aged youngsters are overweight, and 2) around 25 percent of school food is wasted. The new program will provide lower-calorie lunches, more of which—because they will be smaller in size and more varied in contents—will be eaten. In our opinion, smaller waists and reduced wastes are certainly a wise idea.

A popular legend contends that the idea of school lunches was first realized in Munich, Germany in order to reduce the vast number of schoolchildren playing "hooky". In the early 1900's, British law removed the responsibility for feeding school children from charities and made it a governmental duty. Soon after, a number of other countries in Europe followed suit.

In this country, the first successful school lunch program was established in 1894 in Boston and was run mainly by volunteers. It was not until 1935, however, that the government became involved by funneling surplus commodities into the schools. Finally, in 1946, the National School Lunch Act was passed so that there could be federal grants to support school lunch programs. Today, the majority—but not all—of our schools offer a school lunch program.

The typical lunch provided through the National School Lunch Program (the "Type A" lunch) is patterned after the U.S. Department of Agriculture's menu outline. Each lunch should contain the following:

2 oz. meat, poultry, or fish or cheese; or one egg, ½-cup dried beans or peas, or 4 tbsp. peanut butter.
¾-cup of 2 or more vegetables and/or fruit.
1 slice of whole-grain or enriched bread or the equivalent.
½-pint milk.

Unfortunately, many of the commodities used by schools—such as canned vegetables and fruits—are unpopular with children, and hence, often end up in the garbage. Also, the length of the typical lunch "hour" is usually only a half-hour and is cut to around 10 or 15 minutes by the time the students get through the long lunch lines. How fast can little mouths gobble down all of the food in a "Type A" lunch?

A child who is fed properly has a better chance for being a good student than one who is hungry. Obviously, a federally funded school lunch program is an integral component of our country's educational system. But an overweight child is most likely to become an obese adult, one with all of the health problems and decreased life expectancy correlated with excessive body fat. And a child faced with ten minutes to eat an unappetizing and oversized "Type A" lunch will probably not be able to consume it all.

Therefore, offering a smaller school lunch which has more items to choose from will not only save money, but may help to lessen the incidence of both childhood obesity and food waste and emphasize the importance of eating a variety of foods. If students overeat, it certainly will not be to their benefit. And if students simply discard their food, this too cannot be to anyone's advantage.

Instead of protesting the proposed reduction in school lunches, parents, teachers, and other concerned persons should concentrate their efforts on educating children on the importance of proper nutrition, weight control, and regular exercise. Schools should focus on serving appetizing meals, making lunchrooms as appealing as possible, and offering health education to all students. School lunches should set the pattern for lifelong healthy eating habits, and not for overeating, haste, and waste.

FAST FOODS AND THE SCHOOL LUNCH

Fast foods are currently getting increased recognition as an integral component of the American lifestyle. The typical American adult eats in a fast food outlet nine times each month (which is only 10 percent of one's total meals), while the average child or teenager dines on fast foods somewhat more often. There are now more than 300 fast food chains to lure the public and contribute to today's altered food preferences. Who could resist?

"Fast food" may be defined as relatively low-cost food, eaten out of hand, and sold at outlets featuring over-the-counter, fast, convenient service without any frills. Although fast foods have traditionally been available only at restaurant outlets, now hospitals, universities, and school systems are now adopting fast food menus and procedures.

Since the early '70's, a number of school districts around the country have incorporated into their food service the menus and marketing techniques of fast food restaurants. In an attempt to increase food acceptance and decrease food waste, school food service directors have capitalized on the popularity of fast foods among students. Reports indicate that school use of fast foods has increased participation in lunch programs and decreased both food waste and cost per student.

The typical fast food is high in calories, but this is not undesirable for most active, growing children and teenagers. The fiber content of most fast foods is low. This can be compensated for with supplemental coleslaw, tossed salad, vegetables and fruits, all of which enhance the vitamin A and vitamin C contents of the meals as well. Fast foods are generally quite high in sodium (salt), making added salt unnecessary in cooking and at the table. Other minerals, including calcium and iron, can be obtained in significant amounts in various fast foods (calcium from milk and cheese, iron from meat). The protein and B-vitamin contents of most fast food meals are more than adequate. Use of bread or rolls made with enriched flour further improves the nutrient composition of the meals.

Thus fast food school meals can contribute important amounts of protein, vitamins, and minerals to the total diet, along with ample calories and fiber, in a form acceptable to the students and cost-effective for the school system. Since the fast food meals will comprise only one-third of the daily diet during the school week, the proportion of fast foods in the total diet is not undesirably high. Even adding an average of one to three fast food restaurant visits per week, fast food consumption still does not become the major food contribution of the student's diet. And, hopefully, the nutrient value of the non-fast food part of the diet is commendable; this is where comprehensive nutrition education of both students and parents becomes essential.

Obviously, it is preferable for students to eat what they like—especially when their favorite foods are nutritionally significant—rather than have them ignore or abhor their cafeterias, with more Type A lunches found in the trash than in the students.

THE VACATION CHALLENGE

School bells signal the end of school and the beginning of summer with its often carefree habits. When children are home all day, it is very difficult to know what they are eating, but bodies grow in the summer just as they do in the winter and good food is just as important to them.

On vacation it is easy for eating to become haphazard, with hungry children always dropping by the kitchen for an extra bite or two. But a lick and a promise, a bag of candy, a handful of cookies, or a box of crackers are not the solution to a good vacation. Morning, noon, and night, a child's basic food pattern needs to be: a glass of milk, some protein food, some energy food, and fruit or vegetable or both. This meal pattern assures the essentials needed to build muscles and maintain the high energy level needed for a happy, healthful vacation.

The best beginning is a good breakfast. Active play or summer school achievements will not be up to par if children fail to eat a good breakfast, because no child (or adult either) can stay alert all morning long if he has not eaten since the night before.

What is a well-balanced breakfast? A glass of *milk*, but it can be consumed plain, as cocoa, or poured over cereal; *energy food* can be any kind of cereal or bread or roll; breakfast *protein* usually means eggs, bacon, or sausage, but often children like to be different by eating a hot dog, hamburger, or other childhood delicacy at breakfast; and *fruit* can be eaten whole, as juice, or served on cereal. There is no need to have the same monotonous menu day after day. In summer there usually is a little extra time to make breakfast even more of a treat than usual. For instance, how about combining the egg, milk, and energy food in pancakes or French toast or perhaps waffles that can even be made ahead and frozen ready to slip into the toaster for the leisurely breakfast crowd. Remember that variety is often important in maintaining a child's interest in eating breakfast, and many different foods can serve the same purpose, nutritionally speaking.

This same spirit of mealtime adventure can be maintained at lunches and dinners as well during the summer. The pace is relaxed and many children welcome the new experiences that can be gained in the summer when the family can eat and vacation together. They can add to their interest in eating for good health if they have the opportunity to help with some of the food preparation. There is always a great deal of interest in tasting a food that a child has helped to cook!

The keys to good vacation eating are a regular, but relaxed meal pattern and a good bit of physical exercise. It is apparent that parents will need to exercise some initiative in bringing all this about, but the efforts will help their children form good food habits that will lead to the best possible growth and peak capacity for both work and play!

In fact, a summer is long enough to set the stage for the good food habits needed to insure the best scholarly performance when school is in session, too. After all, bodies need good food throughout the year. These ideas apply to teenagers as well as younger children, for teenagers may have a good many hang-ups about good nutrition. In fact, the overweight teenager presents a real problem in modern society.

NUTRITION EDUCATION VS. PRACTICE

Part of the research activities of Harvard's Department of Nutrition has been a cooperative study with the Adolescent Unit of the Boston Children's Hospital to review the eating habits of some overweight youngsters.

One of the most striking observations is how very unhappy these children are. They have extremely unhealthy feelings about food and eating; actually this has become a moral issue with many of them, and they feel it is "wrong" to eat.

While no one in his right mind would wish to ignore obesity in children, or anyone else, it is necessary to keep enlarging our view of the problem if we are going to be able to do something about it.

Research over the past 30 or more years has provided limited knowledge of metabolism in obesity. Information has been sought about the various factors that may lead to obesity, including the physiological controls of appetite. We still don't understand the problem, as is evidenced by the number of teenagers that are overweight. To say the least, our present methods of management of overweight children have been only partially successful. We have *taught* fairly well. Diet histories gleaned from these overweight young people calculate to be perfect 1,000 or 1,200 calorie diets. Yet one youngster actually gained 40 pounds in nine months while proclaiming he was "following his diet."

But enough of this lamentation. Here are a few ideas to follow while waiting for science to unravel the biochemical riddles surrounding obesity.

1. Perhaps treatment should be aimed at *not gaining* rather than losing weight. It is normal for children to grow and to put on weight as they grow. By gradually changing the family picture about food and "good" food habits and attitudes, overwhelming preoccupation with food may then be re-directed into other channels, hopefully active ones.

2. More effort could be directed toward activity—even a study of why some young people "do" less than others.
3. Parents, physicians, nutritionists, and nurses should make every effort to remove the problem of obesity from the realm of moral issues, since over-eating is probably only one side of the fat storage problem.
4. These children should be helped to develop a degree of acceptance of themselves as they are. We learn to live with other dissatisfactions about ourselves—the color of our hair, the shape of the nose, the size of feet. Certainly, a reasonably well-adjusted obese adolescent is a lot easier to work with than a confused and unhappy one.
5. We may need to be a little more discriminating in pronouncing who is really obese. It is entirely possible for a person to be larger than average measurement and have little, if any, excess fat.

At this writing, the sounds of "Pomp and Circumstance" have faded once again and the graduation ceremonies are still recorded within the camera awaiting completion of the roll of film. It seems an appropriate time to write a word to the graduating seniors.

A NUTRITION VALEDICTORY

Today we have a final gift for all of you recent high school graduates. You may have been showered with many presents, but we promise that what we are giving you is unique. Even though we cannot wrap it in ribbons, we hope you will not shove it aside along with other gifts that you will soon forget. What we offer can last a lifetime and be useful no matter what you plan for the years ahead.

Do you suspect we are "members of the establishment" to suggest that advice about food can be all that wonderful? Do you think that good food may be a matter of concern for babies or aging senior citizens, but not for 18-year-olds? Or perhaps you believe that one needs only to eat a strict vegetarian diet (organically grown, of course) to achieve the heights of good health and optimum nutrition. Perhaps you adhere to the idea that you eat when you are hungry and that, when you have had enough, you stop.

But there is much to know about nutrition—much more than previous generations of young people needed to know because so much misinformation is aimed directly at you. If nutrition is bad, it can account for weariness and listlessness, for dull hair, bad skin, flabby muscles, and poor posture. Bad nutrition can lead to poor performance in anything you do, whether it is tennis or typing, football or pingpong, dancing, or working on the job. Perhaps this is a description of someone you know, but we certainly hope you are benefiting from what good nutrition can mean to you. The right food in the right amounts can make all the difference between an attractive and unattractive appearance, can keep weight where it should be, put some valuable zip into work, play, or sports, and can provide a good foundation for health in the far-off future when middle-age catches up, even with you.

Just for an example, can you answer these questions?

1. Does it matter if one skips breakfast?
2. Do young adults need milk, and if so how much is enough and how much is too much?
3. Do grown people need minerals and vitamins, and if so, are there enough in ordinary, everyday foods?

Why can the answers be important to you? Because it has been proven that many young people diminish their productivity by skipping breakfast. It is also known that the body's need for calcium is most easily supplied by dairy products, but that an excess of milk is not desirable because it crowds out other good foods. And everyone, at every age, needs minerals and vitamins, and there are plenty of them in ordinary foods. Yet studies show that all over the United States a great many boys and girls up to the age of 20—so this could mean you—are careless and skimp on the very foods they require.

That is why we say our gift to you today is a chance to change your future. Nutrition can do it, if you will learn to eat a large variety of healthful foods. Every day you need some fruit (including citrus), two or more glasses of milk (or milk plus another dairy product like cheese or ice cream), and some meat, fish, poultry, or eggs. Vegetables, including those that are dark green or yellow also should be a part of the day's foods. Add cereals and breads and other foods to round out your balanced diet and keep you at your right weight. This program, plus a daily dose of brisk exercise, is the package we offer to increase your well-being as you step from high school into adulthood.

Graduation represents a milestone in one's life, and for young women another milestone is reached when they become pregnant and assume the responsibility of eating for the health of their potential offspring as well as for themselves.

A WORD ON NUTRITION IN PREGNANCY

Although diet during pregnancy is extremely important, we will cover this subject briefly with a few general pointers and answers to a couple of questions raised by readers. Our first word of advice is to consult your doctor as soon as you suspect that you are pregnant and then follow his dietary advice carefully. His advice will be far more valuable to you than following old sayings such as the fallacious idea that you are now "eating for two." Remember that an average weight gain during pregnancy is approximately 20 to 25 pounds. Such a weight gain obviously does not give you license to double your food intake during pregnancy, in fact you probably need only about 300 calories more daily during the last six months of pregnancy than you needed prior to pregnancy. Simply adding a couple of important glasses of milk to your daily intake will more than provide these calories unless you drink skim milk.

Another suggestion is that you follow the Basic Four Food Plan (milk, meat, fruits and vegetables, breads and cereals) rather carefully and concentrate primarily on eating nourishing foods. Most expectant mothers will have trouble controlling weight gain if many desserts are a part of the fare.

Vitamin and mineral supplements are of value in some pregnancies particularly when nausea is a recurring problem. Your doctor will prescribe an appropriate supplement if you need one.

One reader wrote that she had read that too much vitamin D during pregnancy may be the cause of mental retardation in some children. She stated that she was pregnant and noticed her obstetrician had provided a vitamin-mineral capsule containing 1,000 International Units of vitamin D. When she showed the article about excess vitamin D to her physician, he told her to keep on taking the capsules. She wrote requesting comments on the use of the capsules.

Upon checking, the news article was full of words such as "potential hazard," "may be," and ended with the sentence, "Reasonable amounts of vitamin D are completely safe, but excessive amounts may be unwise."

Most physicians would agree with that last sentence, thus shifting the question to determining what is a "reasonable amount." To the best of our present knowledge, 1,000 International Units of vitamin D is within the range of reasonable amounts although it is more than is actually necessary. True, you will get some additional vitamin D from certain foods to which it may be added and also from exposure to sunshine, but the amounts from these sources are small and will probably add up to no more than half of what you obtain from a vitamin capsule. When all sources are added together, the total amount of 1500 International Units is still reasonable for an adult including a pregnant woman, although such a level would be on the high side for an infant or young child.

There is no question but that excessive amounts of vitamin D are toxic, but excessive amounts are usually thought of in terms of several thousand International Units taken daily over a period of months. The recommended level of vitamin D for pregnant and lactating women is 400 International Units, the amount that is added to a quart of fortified milk.

Another reader wondered whether women need to be more careful about their calcium intake than men.

The answer is that they do during the last six months of pregnancy and when nursing the baby. Also, after the menopause women are prone to develop osteoporosis (softening of the bones), and so must be very careful not to neglect their calcium foods. At all times, for both men and women, the optimum daily intake of calcium is essential for optimum health. Extra fluoride after the menopause may be prescribed by your physician to help prevent osteoporosis.

MILK: AN IMPORTANT FOOD FOR ADULTS

As adults, it is very easy to tell children how important it is to drink milk so they will grow healthy and strong. Yet many adults who are very conscientious about serving milk to their youngsters fail to drink enough milk themselves.

Although there has been considerable publicity given to the fact that you never outgrow your need for milk, many adults don't really seem to believe that this applies to them. It is easy to understand that children need milk because their growing bones need calcium and phosphorus. These two important minerals, so abundant in milk, are essential to the best possible growth of children; but why should these minerals be needed by adults whose bones are no longer growing? It is hard to realize that bones are continually undergoing change even in adults. Yet this is actually what is happening. The calcium and phosphorus that have been deposited in the bones to give rigidity and strength to your skeleton are constantly being removed from the reserves in your bones and being replaced by new supplies of these minerals. If you drink two glasses of milk daily, you should be absorbing enough calcium and phosphorus to replace the minerals that are being withdrawn. However, the bones will simply become weaker and more easily broken if you do not have enough of these structural minerals in your diet to replace the lost materials. It is wise insurance to regularly drink milk throughout your life. This dietary precaution will help to keep your bones strong at any age.

Perhaps you are thinking to yourself that you really don't care for milk, or maybe you want to approach the idea of milk cautiously because you still think milk is only for little children. If you are skeptical about drinking milk, you may want to start out by using more milk in food preparation. There are many really tempting ways of serving fairly large quantities of milk in a wide range of recipes. For instance, cream soups are very satisfying dishes that accept the flavor of the vegetables in them. You may re-discover the taste pleasure of homemade cream of tomato, cream of mushroom, or other cream of vegetable soups. If you are pressed for time, you may prefer to serve one of the excellent frozen cream soups that are available in the grocery store. These are quick to make and are excellent sources of milk when you dilute the frozen concentrate to its correct strength with milk. You can even add a gourmet touch to the meal by chilling your cream of potato soup to make vichysoisse garnished with a bright sprinkle of chives. For the main course of a meal, milk may be added to the menu by including either a creamed vegetable or a cheese sauce. Even desserts can include a great deal of milk. Applesauce cake or fresh fruit topped with a creamy smooth-stirred custard will surely please you. If you have a blender, there are many milk and fresh fruit combinations to enjoy. By using your imagination, it is a simple matter to include the equivalent of two glasses of milk in your diet each day.

The nutrients needed for good health remain the same throughout life, but the ways of consuming these nutrients required by the body will vary as a person grows, achieves maturity, and then ultimately achieves the status of being a senior citizen. Since these changes in meeting nutritional requirements creep up on us gradually, it is easy to fail to make the necessary adjustments.

Perhaps the most common illustration of this problem is the increase in weight that overtakes many people as they grow older.

FOOD FOR A GOLDEN AGE

"Three score and ten" is no longer a prophecy of dreamers. At the turn of the century the average life span here in the United States was 49 years; today it actually is even more than the proverbial 70. In 1900 our population boasted only three million people over 65; by mid-century this figure was four times as large and has been continuing to climb to more than seven times the 1900 figure.

Yet to simply prolong life is not enough. If the added years are to bring full satisfaction, people must have good nutrition. At 7 months, 7 years, 17, or 70, for maximum well being it is necessary to have an adequate supply of the 50-odd known food nutrients.

So far as is known, food requirements vary very little over the years after one reaches adulthood, with the exception of calories. Energy needs decrease with age and with lessening of activity. Little by little, with each added decade, quantities eaten must be reduced, until by 70 they are about 25 per cent less than at age 25.

Though the total calories are cut, all the other essentials must be included. What older people require is not anything different or elaborate. They do not require special foods, but rather simply enough of the right foods.

Sometimes eating enough of these foods is made very difficult by physical problems like frailty, poor teeth, or other physical handicaps. If these are present, it is important to recognize the problem and do everything possible to correct the situation so that good nutrition is not impossible to achieve.

There are also other difficulties that may lead to poor nutrition. Is there suitable equipment for cooking and is there adequate refrigeration? Is the person doing the cooking a lonely woman who is not interested in bothering just for herself, or is it a man who finds himself face to face with a frying pan for the first time in 70 years? Are grocery stores convenient so that marketing for food is not overwhelming? Are restaurants too far away or too lonely or too expensive? Can small amounts of food be prepared easily and at a moderate cost?

The cost of food for the elderly can be a real problem. Recent statistics show that 75 per cent of the people over 65 have an income less than is calculated to be necessary for maintaining a minimum acceptable level of living. This does not permit wasteful expenditures on special foods or dietary supplements. Yet far too often, hustling salesmen lure those in advancing years into squandering their valuable income on sea salts, sea weeds, bee pollen, or other unnecessary "health foods." False promises of youthful vigor or longer life rob millions of people of millions of dollars which should be spent on food, not frauds.

All that is necessary for optimum nutrition is to spend your dollars wisely on the healthful foods in the grocery store. When fluoride is added to public water supplies, this important nutrient, too, is available at low cost, in the proper amount to help prevent bone deterioration in the elderly.

It is never too early and never too late to establish good food habits. They are basic to health and enjoyment for young and old alike. As we grow older, we can retire from such things as keeping up with the latest rock records or even the nine-to-five-job, but we can never retire from using good sense and judgment in choosing the food we eat. Since more of our citizens are living well beyond 65 years, the health and well-being of the senior citizen is of considerable and growing importance.

QUIZ FOR SENIOR CITIZENS

The process of aging brings about definite changes in our metabolic system. Understandably our knowledge about these changes and how to define them is far from complete. We do know that the aged individual is not the same person he was except just a little older. How well informed are you about nutritional needs after 65?

1. With advancing years, calorie requirements
   a. Increase. b. Decrease. c. Remain the same as in middle life.

Generally speaking, as we age our metabolic rate decreases and our activity decreases, thus reducing our energy or calorie needs. The Recommended Daily Dietary Allowances for a fairly active person indicates approximately a 3.5 per cent reduction in calories per decade. Thus, a 30-year-old woman requiring 2,000 calories per day will need probably some 300 calories per day less when she reaches age 70.

2. As we get older our need for protein
   a. Increases, b. Remains the same as in middle life, c. Decreases.

The protein requirement for the healthy oldster does not seem to be different from that of the younger healthy adult; the recommendation is just under one gram of protein per kilogram of body weight, or 12 to 15 per cent of the total calories.

A practical, enjoyable way to make sure you have the protein you need is to have some animal and some vegetable protein foods in each meal. Milk, cheese, meat, fish, and poultry are the best animal sources. Beans, peas, cereals, and nuts are good vegetable contributors to total protein intake.

3. For the elderly person the levels of minerals and vitamins in the diet should
   a. Be increased over those for the young adult, b. Remain the same, c. Be decreased.

And again, while experimental work in the area of mineral and vitamin needs in old age is rather limited, there does not seem to be evidence supporting an increased need. Actually, it appears at this time that niacin and thiamin could be decreased very slightly because of the somewhat smaller intake of calories in the senior years. Need for iron is reduced in women after menopause.

Occasionally there is evidence of a vitamin or mineral deficiency in the aging population because of factors other than that of changes in requirements. A common cause is lack of funds to provide good nutrition. Another common cause is poor teeth, or even no teeth, with which to chew food. Dental problems among older people certainly add emphasis to the importance of fluoridating community water supplies so that citizens will reap the benefits of fluorides throughout their long lives.

4

THE FOLLY OF FADS

Remember P. T. Barnum, founder of the old Barnum and Bailey circus? He was the master showman of the 19th century, who is credited with the famous phrase, "There's a sucker born every minute." He claimed that the public loved to be fooled, and he made a fortune satisfying that desire.

The public is still paying fortunes for the privilege of being fooled. But today some "Princes of Humbug" may fail to draw the line between innocent amusement and possible fraud. This is especially true in the field of food and nutrition, for tactics similar to those of Barnum can currently be found in many advertisements and stores.

For instance, think of our food supply. Groceries overflow with an unbelievable variety of healthful foods. These foods, full of minerals and vitamins or enriched and fortified when necessary, have helped produce a generation taller and longer-lived than ever before. Moreover, today's foods have conquered yesterday's deficiency diseases such as rickets, beriberi, and scurvy.

Yet these healthful foods are actually denounced as poisonous by Barnum's successors. They make themselves rich by falsely promoting "health" foods and "natural" foods and "organically grown" foods as the key to better health.

The modern day Barnums combine vinegar and honey and claim it will cure arthritis. They take water from the ocean, or even some ordinary grasses, package them, charge a high price, and sell the contents as a cure for cancer, cavities, constipation, or any other human ailment you can name.

Barnum made money by making people laugh. Today's quacks tamper with health. They make every ache and pain sound serious and then sell mysterious remedies to cure the real or imagined illnesses. However, sickness cannot be treated by fake medicines. Any individual who abandons a good diet or a good doctor to follow a fad or a quack is looking for trouble.

Yes, Barnum was right. The public is willing to pay millions for humbug hoaxes, fakes, and fancy phrases, but what if you do not want to go on being hoodwinked?

You don't *have* to be gullible. You can read labels and find out whether the product contains and can do what the ads claim. You can campaign for more adequate governmental regulation and supervision of ads *and* labels.

You can check on the authority. Does he have a real or a fake degree or perhaps no degree at all? Is he telling the truth, or is he misquoting and stating half-truths? Is he up-to-date or are his "reference experts" people who lived and worked 50 years ago? Is he supported by reputable professional organizations?

It is your privilege if you want to go on believing in magic. It won't make you well or keep you forever young, but it will certainly help to make some humbug merchandiser get rich quick.

Medical rip-offs and health quackery cost Americans more than a billion dollars a year, but the cost is even greater when you include the price victims pay in suffering and false hope and in delaying effective medical prevention or treatment. While the days of the traveling pitchmen, with their medicine show from the back of a covered wagon and their magical bottle of elixir appear to be in the past, nevertheless, modern-day quacks abound. They have a firm understanding of the fears and superstitions of potential victims, and they offer very specific and often very scientific-sounding means of curing illnesses and promoting good health. Typical are promoters of "health foods" and vitamin supplements.

Promoters of "health foods" have managed to convince a significant portion of the population that organically grown food is more nutritious and safer than "regular" food; that "natural" is better than "artificial," and that some foods have magical properties. They have built these misconceptions into a new and still-growing form of nutritional rip-off, one which is based on a distortion of the facts about food safety and quality in this country.

First, there is no reason to believe that "organic food" is nutritionally superior. Calling one type of food "organic" is like calling one type of water "wet." An apple is an apple. Altering the way it is grown cannot change its nutritional content. For instance, the amount of ascorbic acid in an apple cannot be made to equal that in an orange by the addition of any amount of chemical stimulant, natural or other. A food's vitamin content is determined genetically. Also, while the "organic" promoter is busy persuading the public that "unnatural" pesticides are dangerous, he is ignoring the very basic fact of life that insects compete with people for food, and that there has never been an authenticated case of illness resulting from pesticide residue on foods purchased at retail stores in the U.S.

Second, while trying to convince people that artificial substances are poisonous, the "health food" promoter will ignore the fact that some of the most poisonous substances known to man occur in natural products; toxins in certain mushrooms, arsenic traces in potatoes, hydrogen cyanide traces in lima beans are examples. The key, of course, is quantity. Enough of a poison from artificial *or* natural sources will kill.

Third, there is no such thing as a magical food. Indeed, ALL foods when eaten as part of a well-balanced, varied diet are health foods. In fact, *the only thing unusually healthy about "organic" foods is the markup on their price.*

Vitamin quacks would have you believe that if a little bit of a vitamin is good, then a great deal of it must be better. The quacks would love to have us all believe that we could benefit from routine vitamin supplementation to our diets.

The fact is that, for most of us, eating moderately from the Basic Four meets all our requirements for vitamins. And it is a fact that considerable danger exists from megadosing vitamin A, vitamin D, and now even vitamin C. The effects of large doses of other vitamins are not well documented, but people who have fallen for the quack sales talk should realize that they are taking part in a large, uncontrolled experiment.

VITAMINS—MYTHS AND REALITIES

Considerable progress has been made in treating and preventing infectious diseases during this century. Many medical mysteries, such as the cause of tuberculosis and the prevention of polio, were made with sudden and decisive advances in medical technology, i.e., the identification of a disease agent or the discovery of a vaccine.

Today, however, health research is extremely complex because chronic physical and mental diseases generally have more than one cause. In this situation where total information on disease causation or prevention is lacking, Americans appear ready and eager to accept any solutions being aired in the popular press. For example, a survey in the 1970's noted that three million adult Americans wore copper or brass jewelry to combat arthritis or rheumatism. About 20 percent of the population believed that arthritis and cancer are due to vitamin and mineral deficiencies. About three-fourths of the population believed that extra vitamins provide more pep and energy. As a society, we seem to be quick to accept any shortcuts to improve our health, despite the lack of evidence.

The human tendency toward gullibility is nothing new, and pseudo-medical fads come and go. The legendary unicorn, that one-horned animal described in Greek mythology, is one appropriate historical example. Filings from the horn of a unicorn were administered as a potion to protect against deadly drugs. Furthermore, those who drank from the horn, according to Greek writers, were protected against convulsions (epilepsy), one of the mysterious afflictions of that day.

Even today, the contemporary counterpart of that early legend is found in the popularity of a potion from the horn of the rhinoceros, a fad which is posing some threat to the species as entrepreneurs seek the raw material on the African scene. A couple of other modern examples of unproven shortcuts to good health are the alleged relationship of food additives and hyperactivity in children and the use of vitamins to cure a wide range of diseases.

Between five and ten percent of all school-age children in the United States have been labeled "hyperactive," or in medical terminology, "hyperkinetic." The hyperactive child is of normal intelligence, but can't sit still and concentrate, with the result that family life is disrupted and havoc may reign in school situations for the child. Many theories on the cause of hyperkinesis have been presented, but none has been proven conclusively. No fully effective treatment exists. As a result, the condition is a terribly frustrating problem both for the young victim and the victim's family.

In 1973, Dr. Benjamin Feingold, a California pediatric allergist, proposed that salicylates (naturally occurring compounds present in many fruits, some vegetables, and several other foods), artificial colors, and artificial flavors are causes of hyperkinesis. He suggested a diet free of these substances as treatment and prevention of the condition. His recommendations have been adopted by the parents of many hyperactive children, and some have reported a distinct improvement in their child's behavior when the diet was followed.

Within the past few years, several careful experiments have been carried out to evaluate the relationship between hyperkinesis and salicylates, artificial food colors, and artificial flavors. We'll take a look at those in a minute, but first we'll describe what is involved in the well-publicized "Feingold diet."

In order to adhere to the Feingold diet and eliminate all the substances he claims affect hyperactivity, all manufactured baked goods, luncheon meats, ice cream, powdered puddings, candies, soft drinks, and punches, as well as tea, coffee, margarine, colored butter, and most commercially produced condiments must be eliminated. Also prohibited are many non-food items such as mouthwash, toothpaste, cough drops, and some over-the-counter and prescription drugs.

Eating in restaurants and school cafeterias is nearly impossible, and convenience foods generally are restricted because they contain artificial colors and flavors. Homemade foods, prepared from "scratch," therefore, become necessary for all family meals. Not only this, but Dr. Feingold strongly recommends including the hyperactive child in the preparation of the special foods and encourages the entire family to participate in the diet program so that the child will not feel "different," his temptations will be reduced, and he will benefit from the positive motivation of team involvement and a group goal.

As you can see, Dr. Feingold's plan focuses total family involvement upon the hyperactive child and requires a substantial commitment of time and energy by the homemaker, as well as participation by siblings and all family members. The program also presents major changes in the family dynamics and activities.

Dr. Feingold claims that, based on clinical observation and testimonials, between 48 and 50 percent of the children who have adhered strictly to his diet program show a marked reduction in hyperactive behavior, and of those who respond, two-thirds do so dramatically. He finds that younger children respond more rapidly and completely than older ones.

Rigorous scientific tests of the Feingold hypothesis, however, do not support his claims. Two types of experimental studies have been conducted; diet cross-over studies and specific challenge experiments. Diet crossover studies involved two groups of hyperactive children, one of which was placed on the Feingold diet for several weeks, and one of which was placed on a diet disguised to look like Feingold's, but actually containing salicylates, artificial colors and flavors. The behavior of the children was observed and tested.

If the behavior was less hyperactive when the children were on the Feingold diet, his theory was supported. Some of these studies have been completed, but the findings have been inconsistent. Some children appeared to improve on the Feingold diet, while others showed no change or worsened. The results gave little support to the Feingold hypothesis, but do not conclusively refute it.

When scientists began to analyze the diet therapy more closely, they recognized the importance of family social pattern change which could also be said to affect the hyperactive child's behavior. It was impossible to pinpoint the diet change as being responsible for the child's improvement.

Specific challenge experiments were devised in an effort to determine whether or not any observed behavioral change could be attributed directly to artificial food colors. Under these experiments, a group of children who appeared to respond to the Feingold diet with a reduction in hyperactivity were selected and divided into a test group and a control group.

Usually there is a second testing phase in which the group assignments are reversed, thus allowing each child to act as his own control. Both groups were fed a diet free of salicylates, artificial colors, and artificial flavors. The test group also had a food that appeared to be within the Feingold guidelines, but actually contained artificial food colors. The control group was fed a food similar in every way, but not containing the additives. The behavior of both groups was observed, tested, and compared. Seven of these studies have been carried out.

One study used almost four times the amount of food color estimated to be the average daily consumption of an American child, and the results showed that scores on a learning test declined slightly after the additives were consumed. Another study used only Yellow Dye No. 5 (tartrazine) and showed no change in hyperactivity. Of the five studies which used the estimated average daily amount consumed, two found a small, but statistically significant increase in hyperactivity after the additives were eaten, and three groups found the additives had no effect on behavior.

These studies do not prove salicylates, artificial colors, and artificial flavors have the dramatic impact on hyperactivity that Dr. Feingold predicted. If artificial colors and flavors are related to behavior, the relationship must be a very small one indeed. The evidence seems to indicate that a few hyperkinetic children, perhaps a fraction of one percent, may experience a mild adverse reaction to one or several artificial colors and flavors in our food supply.

Clearly, the magnitude of any relationship that may exist is so small that changes in child feeding patterns, food processing, and food labeling in an effort to prevent or control hyperactivity are unwarranted and imprudent.

While the Feingold diet is harmless physically and may be helpful therapy in some instances due to its impact on the family, its potential benefits must be weighed against the potentially harmful effect of educating a child to think that his behavior is controlled by what he eats, when this is not proven.

We still have a great deal to learn about the cause or causes of hyperactivity, but we do know now that *the diet by itself is not the answer.* The symptoms of the vast majority of children labeled "hyperactive" are not related to salicylates, artificial food colors, or artificial flavors. The Feingold diet creates extra work for the family and changes the lifestyle—but it doesn't cure hyperactivity. And now, let's look at some questions people ask.

What are salicylates?

Dr. Feingold lists 21 different fruits and vegetables that contain "natural" salicylates, including apples and tomatoes. He also prohibits using any form of aspirin which contains synthetic salicylates. *Synthetic or natural salicylates, the body can't tell the difference.* Salicylates are salt made from a white, crystalline powder which is water-soluble and is used as a preservative.

Can the Feingold diet be harmful?

It could be harmful after a period of time since so many common foods are excluded from the diet. Planning meals to fill the day's nutritional needs could become extremely difficult. Its possible benefits must also be weighed against possible harm from educating a child to think that his behavior is controlled by what he eats, when in fact this is not true.

Lots of people have said the Feingold diet improved the behavior of their hyperactive children. How do you account for this?

The results of Dr. Feingold's early studies have been open to question since the time of their first appearance, partly because he established no control groups in his testing, which is an approach contrary to usual scientific procedures. Consequently, there is no way to know if his positive results were due to elimination of additives, changes in eating habits, increased family attention, maturation or the weather. Subsequent studies have not been able to duplicate Feingold's results.

What do the results of recent studies show?

Recent studies show that if artificial colors and flavors are related to behavior, the relationship is a very small one at best. While a few hyperkinetic children did appear to experience a mild adverse reaction to one or several artificial colors and flavors, the vast majority did not.

Clearly, we still have much to learn about the cause(s) of hyperactivity, but we do know now that diet by itself is not the answer. The symptoms of the vast majority of children labeled "hyperactive" are not related to salicylates, artificial food colors, or artificial flavors. The Feingold diet creates extra work for homemakers and changes the family lifestyle, but it does not cure hyperactivity.

It is up to you. If you are interested in health for yourself and your family, find out what is fact and what is fraud.

You can read material issued by the U.S. Government and by your local and state agencies. The Food and Drug Administration is working to protect *you.*

A SALUTE TO THE FDA

Cracking down on food quacks who are making false claims, catching chiselers who underfill their packages, and condemning unsafe foods. Quite a job!

Yet these are just samples of the many activities of the eagle-eyed people in the Food and Drug Administration. The activities of FDA are reported monthly in a publication called "Enforcement and Compliance."

Patent medicine men have gone modern in the last few years. A number of them appear to be selling odd combinations of vitamins and minerals instead of the old elixirs of life they used to peddle so successfully years ago. One quack claimed over the radio that vitamins cured 53 different diseases as well as prevented nervousness. This is only one type of case where the Food and Drug Administration steps in to fine the offenders and prevent them from making such misleading statements.

Of course, vitamins perform vital functions in the body. **However, beware of a hoax if people try to sell you vitamin mixtures to cure everything under the sun. No vitamin cures cancer, heart disease, or tartar on the teeth. Honest vitamin companies do not make such statements about their products.**

Normal adults who follow the rules of good nutrition do not need extra vitamins from pills. They get plenty of vitamins in the foods that they eat. The rule, "If a little is good, a lot is better," simply is not true for excess amounts of vitamins. *Vitamin capsules which contain amounts far above daily needs are a waste of money.*

In other activities of the FDA, one month's action kept one million pounds of unfit food from reaching the market place! This represents a great deal of money, but it was worth it to help insure the nation's health. Nobody wants a stomach ache from eating some of a bad lot of half-spoiled frozen chicken. Food and Drug Administration inspectors constantly check to make sure that unsafe foods stay off our plates. Many food companies recall and destroy goods which are below standard, even without action by the FDA. By doing this, they keep the reputation of their brands high and their customers loyal.

Most of the food companies try hard to give the consumer a fair value for his money. Food and Drug Administration inspectors keep close tabs on the few cheaters operating in the industry. The trick of printing a higher weight on the label than there is food in the package is an old one which still crops up occasionally. Many consumers will remember the flurry several years ago when it was found that excessive water was being added to some canned hams. There have also been times when the composition of processed meats, particularly weiners, was the subject of much controversy. The legislation controlling the maximum amount of fat legally allowable in hot dogs even managed to swirl to the steps of the White House.

Constant watchfulness means constant safety of our food supply. Hats off to the people at the Food and Drug Administration for the careful job they are doing in keeping our food supply safe and sound.

Our food supply is remarkable not only because of the careful attention it receives via the federal government, but also by virtue of the technological advances resulting from extensive research and development programs funded by private food industries.

ENGINEERING NEW FOODS

Richard E. Lyng, when he served as Assistant Secretary of Agriculture some years ago, presented some stimulating thoughts regarding the role of food engineering at a speech delivered in San Francisco. Part of his speech is reproduced below because we feel he stated the purpose well.

"We are interested in new industry developments in food technology—in the engineering of low cost, nutritious foods. Now available are such products as protein-fortified macaroni, peanut butter, breads, and cakes, flour fortified with lysine, soy-milk formulas, and protein-fortified soft drinks.

"We believe that a properly balanced diet of conventional foods can provide adequate nutrition. Yet we are also aware of changes in dietary habits as well as changes in the nutritional quality of processed foods. Thus, we are interested in 'engineered foods' to the extent that such new foods can offer improved nutrition to the general public. Engineered foods can be defined as those foods which are prepared and processed in ways that improve nutrition, reduce cost, offer greater convenience in meal preparation, improve acceptability, or improve stability. Fortifying or enriching widely used foods would be considered a preferred type of engineering. No opportunity, though, should be overlooked for the useful fortification of any important food. Actually, any engineering which improves the acceptability of a nutritious food and makes it more convenient to use will be a step toward better nutrition.

"We want to see the engineering of foods for nutritional improvement oriented toward better acceptance by the general population through the commercial market. We are not very much interested in foods designed solely for government purchase. In order to achieve improved general nutrition, either through conventional foods or by acceptance of new foods, there will be a need for both government and industry to continue aggressive educational programs to increase public awareness of the need for essential nutrients."

We feel that efforts such as this program by the Food Council of America serve the needs of the public well. However, there is continuous bombardment of "nutrition" information on the public by those who would use the printed word to separate John Q. Citizen from some of his money on the basis of implied threats to health or a magical road to good nutrition that removes the need for any strength of character to achieve it.

BEWARE OF SOME "NUTRITION INFORMATION"

The sorting out of nutrition facts from fads and fallacies is a very difficult job today because you are probably hearing and reading innumerable ideas on the foods needed for good health. Every time you go to the grocery store or drug store today you can expect to find at least one magazine with a reducing diet or other sorts of nutrition information. The American public has a voracious appetite for nutrition information as well as for food. Unfortunately, we usually find that so-called wonder diets proclaiming "you can eat all you want and still lose weight" are far more palatable fare to the buying public than an article outlining a change in overall diet and the need for will power to control weight. We all want to have the easy way to diet success, and we hope to avoid ideas that require effort or seeming deprivation on our part. This attitude leads us to a guideline that will help you in deciding the merit of a food product being advertised for its nutritional value or in determining the worth of articles discussing nutrition.

Guideline number one is: beware of any almost magical claims about food products or diets. There is simply no one food that will provide all the nutrients your body needs. Neither is there any single vitamin or potion that you must buy to be healthy. All the foods you need for good health can be bought in any grocery store. The best possible diet is available to you at the supermarket if you simply know how to select and prepare a good diet. If you are eating right, it is not necessary to take huge capsules stuffed with every vitamin and mineral known to man. No matter how convincing an ad may be, keep in mind that it is not necessary to spend additional money to buy tonics, capsules, and special foods to be healthy. However, it is important to eat a well-balanced diet regularly.

Here is a second guideline to help you. Check the qualifications of the nutritionist who is writing for your consumption. Nutritionists who are qualified to write or speak about your food needs will have an advanced degree (preferably an R.D. or a Ph.D. degree) in nutrition from an accredited and well-recognized college or university. You may be surprised to discover that some pseudo-nutritionists who are informing you about nutrition may not have had any formal education in nutrition. In fact, they may even have bestowed upon themselves an imaginary doctor's degree from a fictitious college or a mail order diploma mill or university. This assumed title of "doctor" does not increase their knowledge of nutrition, but it undoubtedly makes more people listen to them and believe what they are saying. The use of a title that does not rightfully belong to them may be considered fraudulent, but there is no law preventing them from writing about their philosophy of nutrition.

It is apparent, when you read articles written by pseudo nutritionists, that these authors have a sound grasp of human psychology and motivations, although their nutrition information may be distinctly erroneous and is commonly carefully designed to be misleading, but with a ring of authority created by the words used.

Publications by such people are often most interesting to read because they are not tightly bound by any code of ethics to tell only the truth about nutrition. Their writings are typically liberally sprinkled with half-truths or just plain misinformation. The unfortunate thing for the public is that much of this misleading nutrition information is readily available and very convincing. In many cases it leads people to buy expensive, though usually harmless foods and food supplements that strain the budget, but do essentially no physical harm. Unfortunately, in other cases medical treatment that is needed may be delayed while people try food cures that do not treat the problem.

How can you tell if a "health promoter" is a quack?

That's an important question for all consumers. Here are some tips for recognizing the quacks: (1) The quack may be found saying that all our foods are nutritionally bad and that they are "overprocessed, devitalized, and poisoned." (2) They may claim to have an unusual understanding of health and disease and claim that many of the ills of mankind—heart disease, liver disease, kidney disease, poor skin, and others—are due *solely* to poor food. (3) Quite often the quack has something to sell—these days it's usually food supplements or overpriced "natural" foods. (4) They promise quick and sure results, have "testimonials" from "cured" followers to back up their comments and denounce the medical profession and the Food and Drug Administration. Common sense is still a pretty good guide.

Don't you really believe that "natural" has to be safer than processed food?

If we did believe that, then we'd have to believe that raw milk is safer than pasteurized milk, a belief which we clearly do not hold. If you drink raw milk, you increase your chances of developing undulant fever. Also, we would have to believe that everything natural is safe—a belief we do not hold.

There are more than 700 poisonous species of plants in the United States, according to estimates made by horticulturists. The cholesterol in natural eggs may be very dangerous to some people, whereas artificial egg substitutes, without cholesterol, are very safe and may prevent disease for them. Aflatoxins have been shown to cause cancer of the liver in human beings, and they grow quite naturally on some foods, a fact which adds emphasis to the statement that natural foods are not always the safe foods. Nothing is absolutely safe, including some of the most natural substances created by Mother Nature.

One of the common tacks of the food faddist is to promote unusual diets and cloak them in mysticism. Sweeping claims for the merits of off-beat diets often are illustrated by pointing to an individual or group who reputedly have achieved unusual strength, virility, or long life by existing for an entire lifetime on the fad diet currently being promoted. From time to time the Hunzas have been cited by the food faddists.

HURRAH FOR THE HUNZAS?

The Hunzas from a remote mountain region bordering China and Pakistan are frequently said by dyed-in-the-wool faddists to be in superior health because they live largely off whole grains, nuts, and berries. This myth started in the mid-'20s, largely from the non-scientific and hearsay writings of a couple of English food faddists. There is nothing wrong with whole grain cereals, nuts and berries, but neither are they endowed with super-health properties. As for Hunzas, scientific reports corroborating claims for their remarkable longevity and health are only of recent origin and suggest a limited caloric intake, hard work, and an exaggerated food claim.

In 1964 the Morning News of Karachi carried a story about an air lift, called a "wheat lift," that was operating into the remote regions of Hunza, Gilgit, and Skardu. These remote mountainous regions have showy mountain spires and spectacular scenery, but produce little food for the 175,000 people inhabiting these large, but barren expanses.

In addition to the wheat, sugar was also being flown to the Hunzas. To make matters worse from the food faddists' point of view, the sugar was white, which surely must have been a disappointment to those proclaiming the superior health of the Hunzas.

The Karachi article quoted Major Irshad Ahmed, medical chief of the area, as saying that malnutrition was a real problem. There is always a scarcity of meat, milk, and butter. Cherries, apples, and other fruits are plentiful when they are in season, but for at least six months annually, the Hunzas eat "dried fruit, wheat bread, and little else. The incidence of tuberculosis is high."

Thus, it seems that life is rather rigorous in the Shangri La of James Hilton's novel and that the food faddists should pick out another equally remote group of people, but not the Hunzas, to champion their ideas on food and health. Who knows, the Tasaday Manube, a newly discovered tribe in the Philippines who still lives like Stone Agers, may be the next standard bearers for the food faddists. Certainly a tribe that has no knowledge of rice, corn, salt, sugar, or food from the sea will challenge the imagination and creativity of those who would like to create a new diet fad.

Many of the most widely publicized and discussed fads in foods are diets touted as being "the" way to lose weight, seemingly with no pain, strain, or effort on the part of the dieter. Although there are many, many such diets, we will cite just a few of the more popular ones. When you realize that one women's magazine has featured one new diet for weight reduction in each monthly issue, you can easily see that people promoting these diets view them more as parlor conversation than as a means to cure a weight problem permanently.

ABOUT THE PAPAYA

The papaya has received a good bit of notoriety in the past ten years because it has been found to contain papain, which is a proteolytic enzyme. All that the fancy term "proteolytic enzyme" means is that this is a chemical substance that digests, or breaks down protein. Because of this ability of papain, this enzyme has been extracted from papayas and sold to the public as a meat tenderizer. If you sprinkle meat tenderizers on meat, you will notice that the surface of the meat gradually begins to become rather powdery. This is caused by the tenderizer breaking down some of the protein in contact with it into more soluble material. This action, when allowed to continue for an appropriate length of time, results in a more tender piece of meat. With the use of tenderizers, it is possible to purchase less expensive cuts of meat and yet have them acceptably tender when they are broiled or fried. There is no harm to people who eat meats that have been sprinkled with tenderizer, despite the apprehensions that some people have. Meat tenderizers do not have the same action on your stomach that they have on a cut of meat because the enzyme is not able to work in the very acid medium of the stomach.

It is fairly common these days to find advertisements for enzyme preparations, usually from the papaya. It is suggested that these be taken regularly to assist in the digestion of one's food. In particular, the emphasis is on selling items such as papaya extract to people who have digestive discomfort. The inference is that the enzymes that you eat in special enzyme preparations will help your stomach digest the foods by supplementing, or possibly replacing the body's own enzymes. This may sound good in an advertising brochure or magazine. It is almost guaranteed to make numerous perfectly healthy readers begin to worry about the amount of enzymes produced in the body. The gullible are likely to buy such products just as insurance for their digestive enzyme supply. What is not brought out is that enzymes are protein compounds that are quite sensitive to changes in temperature and acidity. When you eat such things as papain or bromelin (the proteolytic enzyme in pineapple), the enzymes will have a very limited action in the mouth. This will be noted when you eat a large amount of fresh pineapple because the tongue may become very slightly sore for a very brief period of time. However, the enzymes are very quickly modified so that they no longer have any capability for digesting protein. The time required for food to travel to the stomach is very, very brief, and the stomach is too acid for the enzymes in any food to maintain their enzyme capability. If you like papayas and pineapple, go right ahead and eat them. We think they are really a treat, too. Just don't count on them to help your body digest the food you eat. Actually, you are fully capable of providing the enzymes needed for normal digestion of food. On a more positive note, the vitamin C content of papaya and other tropical fruits is high. In addition, as you might suspect from the lovely orange color of papayas, the ripe fruit is a good source of vitamin A.

VITAMIN B$_{17}$?

A substance commonly referred to as laetrile or vitamin B$_{17}$ has been in and out of the news frequently in the recent past because this "vitamin B$_{17}$" is touted by some to be a cure for cancer. For years a vociferous few have been arguing that laetrile is an effective means of preventing and curing cancer and therefore should be approved for use in this country. The Food and Drug Administration has barred its use in interstate transactions because of lack of proof of the efficacy of this substance as a cancer cure. However, intrastate matters regarding laetrile are at the discretion of individual states.

Laetrile contains the chemical called amygdalin, derived from the kernels of peaches, apricots, bitter almonds, or apple seeds. These pits are the source of cyanide, a highly dangerous chemical substance because of its toxicity for humans. Supporters, who once claimed that laetrile seeks out cancer cells and releases hydrocyanic acid to kill the cells, now claim that cancer prevention and cure are dependent on laetrile treatment, and that laetrile treatment should be legalized. Once again, we will present testimony from one user. W. A. Nolan, author of "A Doctor in Search of a Miracle," tells the following true story:

Dr. Nolan saw a patient he calls "Mary"—a 35-year-old mother of three children, who was pregnant with her fourth child. Her examinations revealed that she had an early case of cancer of the uterus. Dr. Nolan wanted to put her in the hospital immediately and begin treatment, but he was unable to do so.

As her husband later told the story, Mary did begin to make plans to enter the hospital right away, but before she began her treatment, she talked with a friend who spoke of another woman who supposedly had the same disease as Mary. She had gone to a clinic in Mexico, just below the Texas border, where she had been given laetrile. According to Mary's friend, this cleared everything right up, without radiation, surgery, or anything else.

Although Mary was a sensible woman, the idea of either surgery or X-ray of her uterus frightened her, so she insisted on giving this other method a try before returning to Dr. Nolan. For a while after returning from Mexico, it seem that she was getting better. The spotting symptoms that had caused her to seek medical treatment in the first place disappeared, and Mary and her husband were convinced that the $3,000 they had spent for the "Mexican treatment" was worth it.

Mary believed she was cured. Six months later, she was bleeding every day and losing strength fast. She then realized that the laetrile had been useless. When she returned to Dr. Nolan, the cancer had grown to the walls of the pelvis on both sides and had infiltrated the bladder from the front and also the rectum. There was no longer any effective treatment available. She died within a month. This true story is from "A Doctor in Search of a Miracle", authored by William A. Nolan.

Dr. Thomas Jukes of the University of California at Berkeley wrote "Laetrile for Cancer," an article appearing in the *Journal of the American Medical Association* (Sept. 13, 1976). He noted that Laetrile is "another chapter . . . in the melancholy history of cancer quackery," adding that this chapter follows the outline of its predecessors:

"First, a remedy is introduced resulting from a novel 'strange idea.' Next, its promoters become so dedicated to advocating the remedy that they cannot retreat from a position which becomes untenable as a result of exposure of the worthlessness of the remedy. Third, the promoters are reinforced in their fraudulence by champions of the 'underdog' against the establishment, and by the surviving relatives of deceased victims of cancer. These relatives, because of feelings of guilt, cling to the belief that treatment with the 'remedy' was the best possible therapy.

"Finally, vast sums of money and amounts of time are wasted on elaborate tests of the 'remedy' by qualified scientists who should be doing something useful. These tests usually are undertaken because of coercion by legislators and other governmental officials who respond to letters from voters—letters that often are generated by the 'health food' press."

The FDA decision to permit clinical trials of laetrile followed more than a year of effort on the part of the National Cancer Institute to persuade them. The NCI claimed that the trials were necessary to settle the long-lived debate over whether laetrile has any effect upon cancer, or whether it is, in fact, a fraud.

The January 28, 1982 issue of the *New England Journal of Medicine* contains a report on a major study "closing the book on laetrile." The trial was conducted with support from the National Cancer Institute and concluded that laetrile simply does not work—even in combination with the special diets and vitamin supplements promoted by some laetrile advocates. In a group of nearly 200 cancer patients—who were in generally good condition but in the advanced stages of the disease—laetrile treatment showed no beneficial effects, and several patients had symptoms of cyanide toxicity.

Following the journal article, a *New York Times* editorial pondered over the reasons for laetrile's popularity in spite of the fact that it was never shown to be effective and exists merely as a dangerous health fraud. The *Times* felt that laetrile represents a lack of communication between physicians and the public. In examining the question further, we can see that the success of laetrile also represents the inability of the news media to convey accurate medical information. Opting for sensationalism over fact, the news media often feed the public outright health fraud—in megadoses.

Responsibility for amending the laetrile hoax and other such fraudulent situations lies in three laps:

1. The scientific/medical/nutritional community needs to educate the news media and the public in terms understandable to all;
2. The news media should assist the public to separate fact from fraud; and
3. The public must opt for scientific truth over magical myths despite the lure of the latter.

With today's ecology fad and a strong movement to return to nature, there has been a great flurry about "natural" foods. To some people, anything that has undergone any processing is totally unfit to eat. In their eyes, so-called natural foods are bountifully endowed with some nutritional attributes that would surprise even Mother Nature herself.

MOTHER NATURE'S BOUNTY?

It seems the best way to put such items as refined sugar, brown vs. white-shelled eggs, wheat germ oil, brewer's yeast, and cider vinegar into perspective is to answer some questions that have been gleaned from across the nation.

My husband and I have done a little investigating in the world of food, and there is one major point on which we cannot agree. I wonder if you could arbitrate. Since cane sugar supplies little except energy to the body, my husband maintains that it can be cut out from the diet entirely. Instead, he believes in substituting simple sugars such as honey or corn syrup. He thinks that simple sugars are appreciably easier to digest and use and, therefore, much better for the body. I maintain that a certain amount of cane

sugar (as in a dessert once a day or in making muffins, etc.) won't do any harm. I also maintain that cane sugar isn't very hard on the digestive system.

You know more nutrition than your husband. Your ideas are perfectly correct. The utilization of cane sugar is very simple for the body and there is little difference in the ease of digesting honey, corn syrup, and cane sugar. None of these is difficult to digest.

What is a natural sugar and what does it do for you? In what foods are natural sugars found?

All sugar is "natural" in that it is made in nature by some living plant, for example, sugar cane or sugar beets, most fruits, or by a living animal, i.e., the honey bee. For commercial purposes, the sugar of cane and beets is concentrated and refined, ending up as ordinary granulated or powdered sugar. Unrefined sugar, as in raw honey or brown sugars, is often referred to as natural sugar. Any type of sugar has essentially the same nutritive value; each is basically a concentrated source of carbohydrate and will provide calories for energy. The nutritive contribution of the impurities in the so-called natural sugars is too small to be of any consequence in the amounts normally consumed.

Would you please let me know if brown eggs are better than white? My husband insists there is a difference, so I buy brown eggs.

The color of egg shells has nothing to do with the nutritive qualities of eggs. Eggs are good food, the white being high in protein, and the yolk being a good source of fat, many of the B vitamins, and minerals, particularly iron. The yolk is also a concentrated source of cholesterol in a readily absorbable form, so on low cholesterol diets the intake of egg yolks should be limited to one or two per week. The intake of white, since they do not contain cholesterol, need not be limited in this way.

Will dried brewer's yeast or any so-called health foods help to cure my lack of energy?

Not unless your lack of energy relates to some nutrient lack in your diet which will be supplied by the yeast or health food; if this is the case, a varied diet providing good nutrition and made up of foods purchased at any grocery store will do equally well at less cost. All grocery stores today are "health food stores" because all foods contribute to health.

I suffer with arthritis and have been advised to take honey. What is your opinion?

Honey is a pleasant-tasting food, essentially sugar, but it is of no value in the treatment of arthritis or other diseases. However, do not hesitate to eat it and enjoy it for its sweet taste and its calories for energy.

I was told that apple cider vinegar was good for arthritis. Is this true?

It is not true.

I have heard that amino acid in liquid form and lipids made from soy, rice, and wheat germ oils are supposed to increase energy and endurance. Is this true? This preparation is rather expensive, and before I try it I would like to know your opinion. Is there any cheaper substitute I could take? I am 70 years of age.

Amino acids in liquid form are no better from a nutritional viewpoint than those in roast beef, sardines, or hamburger and they don't taste nearly as good. The lipids from soy, rice, and wheat germ have no unusual energy or endurance properties not possessed by other edible fats or oils. A cheaper substitute for the concoction you are describing is an ordinary, well-balanced diet. How do you think you got to be 70 years of age—living off liquid amino acids?

With the tightening of the economy, the problem of managing the family income as widely as possible without sacrificing good nutrition is of interest to all. Frequently mothers and wives worry that they are not providing adequate amounts of vitamins in the food they serve their families. They may feel that vitamin capsules are necessary "insurance" so they can be certain nothing is lacking.

TO SUPPLEMENT OR NOT TO SUPPLEMENT?

With all due respect to Shakespeare, we would like to paraphrase the famous quotation from Hamlet and ask "To supplement (with vitamin capsules) or not to supplement? That is the question."

You may have noticed when you have been in a drugstore that vitamin supplements can be a pretty expensive item, even when you buy them in the large, economy-size bottle. With the ever-increasing cost of living, most of us are concerned with trying to be well-nourished and comfortably well fed without spending money on unnecessary items. You have probably asked yourself if those vitamin supplements really are necessary to good health or can you afford not to take them. The answer is dependent on your customary dietary habits and the state of your health. If you are in good health and are eating a varied diet as outlined by the Basic Four Food Plan, you should not need to take a vitamin supplement. The Basic Four Food Plan includes two or more glasses of milk each day for adults, two or more servings of meat or meat substitutes, four or more servings of enriched or whole grain bread and cereal products, and four or more servings of fruits and vegetables. The four or more servings of fruits and vegetables should include a citrus fruit every day and a dark green, leafy vegetable or a yellow one at least every other day. This plan provides a wide variety of food and includes foods that are high in the nutrients needed for good health.

Now, as we all know, it is one thing to know what you need to eat, and it may be quite another matter for you to actually eat it. If you are to fairly decide about your diet and what it does for your health, you will need to be really honest with yourself. Do you regularly drink your two glasses of milk (or eat other dairy products or foods containing large quantities of milk or cheese) or do you just get the milk occasionally? Are you a chronic breakfast skipper who rarely includes a citrus fruit in the diet? Are you one of these people who loathes vegetables and rarely eats them? Or are you one who specializes in meat and potatoes, with little else to eat? Take a close look at how you normally eat and then you can determine whether or not vitamin supplements might be a good idea for you or someone in your family. If you find that you and your family are regularly eating a good diet, you might as well reward yourself by taking the money that would be spent for a vitamin supplement and buy something you would really enjoy. On the other hand, if your dietary pattern is not what it might be, it is either time to make a significant change so that your food intake supplies the nutrients you need or else you should consider taking a vitamin supplement. It really is far better to reform your habits than it is to take a vitamin supplement because foods contain minerals, protein, fats, and carbohydrates as well as just the vitamins found in capsules.

There are some people who may need a vitamin supplement. Young babies benefit from a vitamin supplement which their doctors will prescribe. Persons with food sensitivities may sometimes need to take a vitamin and/or mineral supplement to replace nutrients in the food which had to be removed from the diet. This is particularly true if the food sensitivity is due to milk. However, if you are sensitive to something like strawberries or chocolate, there is no need to be concerned about supplementing with vitamin pills.

MEGAVITAMIN THEORY

There are many people, even some physicians, who claim that daily high doses of water-soluble vitamins will treat and prevent such conditions as the common cold, hypercholesterolemia, senility, and schizophrenia. Dr. Linus Pauling, the distinguished chemist and twice the recipient of a Nobel Prize, is the theoretician who coined the term "orthomolecular." He argues that much illness is a consequence of having a disordered molecular environment within the body and that restoration of this environment can be achieved by an individually determined regimen of vitamin supplements. There are enough big words in the megavitamin theory to make it sound impressive to some people.

However, consider a number of points before you run out and stock up on vitamins. First, Dr. Pauling is not a physician nor a nutritionist. Second, his advice is nothing new. Actually, the "megavitamin theory" became popular among health faddists in 1953, 15 years before Pauling offered his "new theory." Third, in the past 15 years, megavitamin therapists have refused to conduct controlled clinical studies on the grounds that they "know" the treatment works, and it would be unethical for them to withhold treatment from their patients. An American Psychiatric Association Task Force, established in 1973, evaluated the theory and practice of megavitamin therapy in schizophrenia and concluded that the basic science on which the theory was based was inconsistent and contrary to established biochemistry.

By discriminating about these new "diet theories" and, in the meantime, eating a well balanced diet, you can be well nourished. Massive doses are not necessary.

What is considered a large amount of vitamin C?

Minimum body requirements for vitamin C (ascorbic acid) under normal conditions of health are rather small, around 10 to 20 milligrams per day. Thus, ascorbic acid taken in pills on a daily basis of 500 milligrams or more can certainly be considered large quantities. Diets that include a citrus fruit or juice, or tomato juice, provide 70–80 milligrams per day—clearly an adequate intake.

Since vitamin C is water-soluble, doesn't this indicate that amounts exceeding that which is needed by the body are excreted?

In general, this is true, but may not apply to such high levels as 10,000 to 20,000 milligrams daily.

In what ways can vitamin C in large quantities adversely affect health?

Toxic effects of abnormally large amounts of vitamin C that have been reported include renal stones, gastrointestinal disturbances, sensitivity reactions, conditioned need for large amounts of vitamin C, and destruction of vitamin B_{12}.

Can these be serious medical problems?

They may well be. Some of them have been verified to be problems with persons who already are suffering from certain medical problems.

What are some of the more common reactions resulting from habitual ingestion of large amounts of vitamin C?

Gastrointestinal disturbances, such as nausea, abdominal cramps, and diarrhea are, perhaps, the most consistent reactions noted. These may be due to the ascorbic acid itself or to allergic reactions, such as hives, swelling, and skin rashes.

What is meant by "conditioned need"?

This refers to the reports that certain persons, after prolonged intake of 2,000 to 3,000 milligrams (mg) of extra dietary ascorbic acid, developed scurvy (as extreme vitamin C deficiency) when they ceased taking the extra ascorbic acid. That is, humans, who had been perfectly healthy with normal amounts of vitamin C in foods, became conditioned to require huge amounts to maintain normal health. This conditioning may extend to the infants of mothers who take large amounts of vitamin C during their pregnancies. There was one report of two infants who developed scurvy, presumably because of this situation.

Is there any scientific explanation for ascorbic acid dependency occurring after prolonged consumption of excessive amounts of vitamin C?

It is believed that the human body protects itself against excessive amounts of vitamin C by destroying the extra vitamin C when large amounts are ingested. Apparently, this mechanism continues after vitamin C has been reduced to normal amounts, so that signs of vitamin C deficiency appear.

How can large amounts of vitamin C interfere with another vitamin in the body?

Thousands of complex interactions take place continually within the human body, most of them still unexplained by scientists. Two researchers have actually demonstrated the destruction of vitamin B_{12} by large amounts of ascorbic acid.

Is there any beneficial effect from large dosages of vitamin C?

Among the many claims made about the value of large amounts of ascorbic acid, the ones concerning prevention and treatment of the common cold have aroused the most attention. There are many anecdotes about vitamin C and its benefits in this regard, but these anecdotes do not prove that vitamin C in excessive amounts can be valuable in regard to colds. Some well-controlled studies have shown minor differences on number of days away from work, but the general practice of dosing oneself with large amounts of vitamin C is highly questionable.

Does a person require more vitamin C during infections or other illnesses than at other times?

People may need greater amounts of vitamins during periods of ill health, but the amounts are relatively small in comparison with the large doses of vitamin

C currently being taken by some persons. Therapeutic measures under these conditions are approximately 100 to 200 mg per day, far less than the 500 to thousands that have been shown to have the possibilities of being toxic.

Shouldn't I take extra vitamins to keep myself healthy?

Not unless you have a vitamin deficiency. If you are eating a balanced diet, all the vitamins necessary to ensure good health will be found in your food and in a form far more pleasant and less expensive than in a pill bottle.

Will it hurt me to take extra vitamins, just in case I need them?

It might not hurt you, but it might! It will certainly hurt your pocketbook. Although the excesses of the water-soluble vitamins, B and C, are naturally excreted by the body (it is said that the richest source of vitamins is the New York City sewage system), nevertheless, it is possible that diarrhea, kidney stones, reduction of female fertility, and a certain type of vitamin dependency can develop along the way. In the case of the fat-soluble vitamins, A and D, overdoses can cause serious damage. A number of deaths and cases of unnecessary surgery have been recorded as directly related to either taking high-potency preparations, combining too many different kinds of supplements, or taking more than the recommended dosage.

What about vitamin E? Lots of people are adding that to their diets, aren't they?

Vitamin E is essential to good health, but it is not the cure-all vitamin that health food stores would like you to believe. Vitamin E is so plentiful in foods we eat (vegetable oils, whole grains, leafy vegetables) that it is almost impossible to develop a deficiency if you are eating a well-balanced diet. Yet, because of a myriad of undocumented claims for its curative powers, vitamin E sales continue to expand, and this has health scientists very much concerned. They deplore the widespread fascination with vitamin E, warning that people supplementing normal diets with vitamin E are taking part in massive, uncontrolled experiments. If a deficiency in vitamin E creates a disorder that can be cured by adding vitamin E to the diet, it cannot then be assumed that adding vitamin E will *prevent* the disorder. Instead, it must be assumed that added vitamin E, taken particularly in large amounts, is likely to cause another disorder! Until this vitamin is understood better in terms of its role in health and its potential toxicity, vitamin E still can be described as "a vitamin looking for a disease."

A few people have become overly concerned with the importance of vitamin A. Of course, vitamin A is essential to the maintenance of normal health and performs several invaluable roles in the body. However, this vitamin, as well as vitamin D, are stored by the body. Harmful effects have been noted when large capsules of these vitamins are taken frequently over an extended period.

HYPERVITAMINOSIS A

When a person consumes very, very large quantities of vitamin A over a long period of time, he or she will gradually develop an impressive sounding condition known as hypervitaminosis A. It takes time to build up such a high level of vitamin A in the body. One huge dose will not cause you to develop the symptoms.

Vitamin A is stored in the liver, a fact that explains why you can gradually build up a toxic level of this vitamin if you regularly take large doses of it. The ordinary diet is far from dangerous in its vitamin A content. In fact, it appears that about the only food that could cause you to build up too much vitamin A in your body is polar bear liver, and how many people do you know who eat polar bear almost exclusively? In other words, there is almost no possibility that you will have too much vitamin A in your diet. The actual fact is that you are far more likely to have too little vitamin A unless you are careful to eat a dark green, leafy or a yellow vegetable at least every other day. If this is the case, why is there reason to be concerned about a toxic level of vitamin A?

You will find that there are fairly inexpensive capsules of vitamin A that can be purchased without a prescription. The difficulty begins to arise when people buy the capsules of vitamin A containing 25,000 International Units of the vitamin in each one. When you realize that the recommended daily allowance is only 5,000 International Units of vitamin A, it is apparent that even one of these large capsules of vitamin A is five times more than the normal individual needs. As if that were not a large enough overdose, some well-intentioned, but over-zealous people will take two of these capsules every day. If an intake of 50,000 International Units of vitamin A is taken regularly, you will soon build up an abnormally high level of vitamin A in your liver, and it will take you several days or even weeks for this level to return to normal after the vitamin A supplement is discontinued. Fortunately, there are symptoms that occur as the vitamin A level begins to build to a toxic dose, and these symptoms often will cause people to consult a doctor who can then effectively treat the patient. Early symptoms of hypervitaminosis A include nausea, depression, and loss of appetite. These symptoms will continue until the vitamin A level is decreased. In children, hypervitaminosis A is a particular concern because it can lead to mental retardation in very severe cases.

Since these problems have been noted, the practice of giving large doses of vitamin A to pregnant women has been discontinued by most people. It is hoped that the FDA will soon limit Vitamin A capsules that can be purchased without a prescription to 10,000 I.U. or less.

ORGANIC WINDMILLS

Don Quixote and his legendary jousting with imaginary windmills is somewhat reminiscent of the present furor over "organic foods." The contemporary trend toward the natural life of earlier years has invaded the food supply system in a number of ways, including efforts to return to farming without chemical fertilizers and pesticides. Considerable emotion has been invested in attempting to obtain legal definitions of "organic foods" and other related legislation.

As a consequence of the public clamor, the U.S. Department of Agriculture created a study team on organic farming in 1979 to study the potential contributions of organic farming and to satisfy consumer demands for more comprehensive data on organic farming technology. Our guess is that the latter reason was by far the dominant factor in the study.

This study relied on a variety of sources of information, including 69 organic farms in 23 states, a Rodale Press survey of *The New Farm* readers, interviews and correspondence with organic farmers and their spokesmen, and literature reviews and two study tours abroad.

False fears about chemical fertilizers, nutrient-depleted soils and about pesticides have mainly been responsible for the search for unconventional, yet productive farming methods. Unfortunately for the fearful consumer, foods produced by so-called "organic" farms supply neither improved health nor guaranteed super nutrition.

In fact, many organic farmers find that they have to use some synthetic fertilizers and herbicides in order to produce edible products. And organic food almost always will cause higher costs than are incurred when regular produce is purchased.

The organic farming movement encompasses a wide range of philosophies and practices. This is mainly due to the fact that there exists no legal definition for the term "organic" at the national level. In both a scientific and a dictionary sense, all foods are organic because all foods contain the element carbon and all are derived from living organisms (plants and animals). Thus, as it stands now, the term "organically grown" can mean whatever the merchant wants it to mean unless the state in which it is grown and marketed has a legal definition of the term.

As Peter Barton Hutt, formerly of the Food and Drug Administration once said, "It's very simple to put a sign over some raw produce and say 'organically grown'. Who in heaven's name will ever be able to figure out whether it is or it isn't? Who's going to test it; who's going to make sure it's not inaccurately labeled?"

Obviously, there is much room for fraud. Even the honest organic farmer can end up with pesticides in his produce because residue chemicals from nearby farms can be deposited by wind and water and are nearly impossible to avoid.

The real problem is the lack of a legal definition of organic farming. The USDA Study Team on Organic Farming defined it as, ". . . A production system which avoids OR LARGELY EXCLUDES the use of synthetically compounded fertilizers, pesticides, growth regulators, and livestock feed additives. To the maximum extent feasible, organic farming systems rely upon crop rotations, crop residues, animal manures, legumes, green manures, off-farm organic wastes, mechanical cultivation, mineral-bearing rocks, and aspects of biological pest control to maintain soil productivity and tilth, to supply plant nutrients, and to control insects, weeds, and other pests."

Thus, even this recent USDA study included as "organic" those farms where synthetic fertilizers and pesticides were used. The study also stated that these farmers consider themselves to be organic farmers. Would YOU consider paying increased prices for these so-called "organic" farm products?

The report concluded that many organic farmers perform in commendable fashion, utilizing cost-efficient, energy-saving soil and crop management techniques. The Study Team felt, however, that the future prospects for large-scale organic farming are limited. Significant changes would have to be made in the overall structure of the U.S. agricultural system. Consumers would have to learn to do without the variety of foodstuffs now available.

It is estimated that if the use of pesticides alone were banned in the U.S., crop losses would reach 50 percent, and food costs would increase four or five times! If we depended on human labor to replace the need for pesticides, it is estimated that it would require 17.7 million people working for six weeks to remove all the weeds from the U.S. cornfields; if people worked a 48-hour week at $3.00 per hour wages, this would be equivalent to over 100 percent of the value of the entire U.S. corn crop.

Environmental regulations in this country could also create serious food problems abroad, especially in the developing nations where crop losses, even with pesticides, are often substantial.

Organic foods are not higher in nutritive value than commercially-grown products. Psychologically, the food you grow yourself may seem tastier and healthier than what you buy in the local supermarket, but any claims for the nutritional superiority of organically-grown foods are not substantiated. The USDA Study Team on Organic Farming supported this fact. So, if you are paying extra money for organic foods in order to obtain extra nutrients, you are only adding to your food bills and not to your nutritional status.

The USDA Study Team on Organic Farming recommended that new research and educational programs on organic farming be developed. However, we may be better off, both money-wise and health-wise, in expending our efforts on the establishment of a legal definition for "organic" and "organic farming," the development of technological advances in agriculture, and the education of the public on the facts about nutrition and health. This requires a combined effort by government, scientists, and health educators. Results could be far more encompassing than those derived from the limited surveillance of a self-defined agricultural group.

Personally, we resent taxpayers' dollars being used by the USDA for investigating the possible merits of organic farming and supporting two junkets to Europe by the study team. Countless research studies over the past 40 years have demonstrated that organic farming has no practical value in large scale farming, and so-called "organic foods" are just another ploy in the ornamentation of the professional food faddist and health huckster.

Can organic foods provide as nutritious a diet as ordinary foods?

First, let's define "organic": All foods are organic because they contain carbon. You are probably referring to "organically-grown foods," which are those foods grown with organic fertilizers, such as manure and composts, rather than chemical fertilizers. Presumably, no pesticides or insecticides were used during the growing of the foods. However, pesticide residues have been found on "organic" foods, sometimes in greater amounts than on foods not labeled "organic"!

Don't worry, though—the amounts of pesticide residues found on either types of foods have been so small as to be insignificant to anyone's health. For that matter, there has been no documented case where pesticide residues on foods purchased in any store in the U.S. have caused illness in human beings.

Organically-grown foods are nutritionally equal to ordinary foods, but they are *not* superior. They usually are more expensive, and the quality from a sanitary and aesthetic view is not as good. The apples may have worms and the vegetables more bugs, and the raisins may have more bits of stems to get in your way while munching.

The secret to good nutrition, for adults and for children, is to consume a variety of foods and to eat no more than you need to maintain desired weight. Within this variety, it is perfectly acceptable to include organically-grown foods if you wish to spend your money this way.

Although there is much more that could be said about various fads and nutrition misinformation bombarding the public, we will wind up with a short nutrition quiz for your amusement or amazement.

QUIZ YOURSELF

From the earliest of recorded history, people have attached myths of fancied and supernatural powers to foods. Every culture had had its particular list of food taboos and foods thought to be particularly valuable. Time has proven most of the ideas to be unwarranted. However, some have been shown to have had a bit of truth in them.

We know now that when a food demonstrates value in a particular disease, it is because of a specific nutrient. Thus, limes (or lemons) cured scurvy. Now we know it was the vitamin C they supplied. An ancient treatment for goiter was dried or burned sponge, a rich source of iodine. Can you sort out the facts from the fallacies in this nutrition quiz?

1. Some foods, when eaten together, are poisonous or harmful:
   a. Milk and fish, b. Milk and orange juice, c. Milk and cucumbers,
   d. Ice cream and lobster

Answer: No evidence indicates that combinations of foods are poisonous. Foods themselves are combinations of nutrients. Perhaps in the days before refrigeration, by coincidence, several people ate milk with fish that wasn't fresh enough and got sick. If you don't drink milk with fish because of this idea, do you eat fish chowder, oyster stew, or filet of sole bonne femme? And if you fear milk and orange juice, how do you feel about orange sherbet, orange floats, and orange puddings? If you worry about lobster and ice cream, perhaps you are wise, but not because of the combination, but because of the large amount of food this implies.

2. There are foods which have specific value for certain bodily functions:
   a. Yogurt helps keep one young, b. Fish and celery are brain foods, c. Carrots are good for the eyes, d. Beets build blood, e. Red meat makes you strong

Answer: As for this list, yogurt or any other fermented milk product has no spectacular power. It is no better than the milk from which it is made. While fish is a fine food that is rich in good protein, and celery is a pleasant vegetable, there is no evidence that, after they are eaten and digested, the brain cells or any other cells can differentiate between nutrients from these foods in preference to the same nutrients from other foods.

In a sense, carrots are good for the eyes, but not because they are carrots, but rather because carrots contain a lot of carotene, a substance readily changed into vitamin A in the body.

Beets are not a good source of any of the nutrients considered necessary for the formation of blood.

Meat does provide many valuable nutrients, is very satisfying and pleasant to most of us. However, the same nutrients can be obtained from other sources.

3. Lots of us have specific ideas about foods. Can you separate the facts from the fancies:
   a. Honey isn't fattening, b. Toast has less calories than bread, c. Vegetable fats are lower in calories than animal fats, d. White shelled eggs are better than brown, e. Synthetic vitamins are harmful, f. Vitamin deficiency causes gray hair, g. Vitamin B_{12} cures breaking hair and splitting nails

Answer: There are no facts in this entire list. Honey is high in sugar and sugar, regardless of its source, furnishes four calories per gram (16 for each teaspoon). Of course, a little bit of honey or any other food is not fattening. The *amount* eaten is the important factor.

Toast is bread with some of the water removed and some of the starch dextrinized. The calories are still there unless part of the bread gets stuck in the toaster. Remember, water does not furnish calories.

Fat is fat regardless of its source. Vegetable fats differ from animal fats in chemical makeup, but *not* in calorie value.

The color of an eggshell is a function of the breed of the chicken and has nothing to do with the nutritive value of the contents of the shell. Any imagined difference must be due to aesthetic implications.

There is no difference between synthetic vitamins and those occurring naturally in foods. They are identical.

Gray hair is not caused by a lack of any known vitamin in the diet, and addition of vitamins or any other dietary supplement will not prevent it.

Vitamin B_{12} is clearly an essential nutrient and is a specific treatment for pernicious anemia, but its absence from the diet has no relation to breaking hair or splitting finger nails. Both hair and nails, like other body tissues, are dependent on good nutrition and may be impaired by a poor diet, but these two problems are not known to be related to faulty diet.

4. Some of the food advertisements, while not inaccurate, can be misleading. How are you in judging the value of some of these well-known claims?
   a. Margarine made the "Danish" way is never hydrogenated. b. Diet bread has only 46 calories per slice, but is high in minerals and vitamins and will help the weight watcher in his fight against too many calories.
   c. Buy our bread. It is now made with polyunsaturated fat.

Answer: The claims in this advertisement are perfectly true, but the implication is that there is something wrong with hydrogenation (the process by which liquid oils are solidified). Margarines made of vegetable oils that are solid at room temperature, such as coconut oil, contain large amounts of saturated fatty acids. In other words, the oil is naturally hydrogenated—no need to do it artificially.

This statement is also true, but unless you think pretty carefully, you might be misled into thinking this is really a calorie-saving product. A slice of regular bread supplies 60 calories; the diet bread has 46. You are paying more for less. Also, one is apt to think that, since it is "diet" bread, it is possible to eat all you want and not get fat. That, of course, is not true.

This ad is really stretching things to make a sales pitch. Do you know how much fat there is in one slice of regular bread? One-seventh of a teaspoon or 0.7 grams of fat. In amounts that small, it makes little difference whether the fat is saturated, unsaturated, animal, or vegetable.

5

WHAT IS SAFE TO EAT?

The American consumer is deluged today with stories about the terrible things found in foods, from DDT, to mercury, to lead, DES, PCB's, ad infinitum. The long parade of warnings is probably just beginning. Tomorrow it may be gold, cadmium—who knows what? In part this is because scientific techniques to analyze foods have improved greatly in recent years, and one can now find traces of almost anything in anything!

On many sides one hears the question, "Is any food safe to eat?" The answer is an emphatic *yes*. All foods as normally marketed in this country are safe to eat, assuming they are properly prepared, clean and wholesome, and that includes fish, all kinds of fish.

For years we and many others have been teaching about the fine nutritive qualities of fish and its value as an important part of diets designed to lower the cholesterol level of the blood and hence help prevent or postpone the onset of our commonest type of heart disease. The discovery recently of mercury levels in some tuna and much swordfish that exceed the Food and Drug Administration interim guidelines has sent a panic wave through the ranks of many who ought to know better. Personally, this arbitrary guideline appears to be drawn at least twice as low as it can be. Ask your doctor when was the last time (or first) that he has seen or heard of ill health of any kind where the mercury content of fish was the cause or even suspected cause? Write your local or state medical society, your city or state health department, or the United States Public Health Service, and ask the same question. It is a safe bet that the answer will be "never."

The fact is that fish are safe to eat, all fish. What is unfortunate about all this is that 600,000 Americans die annually from heart disease, but there has never been a symptom of injury, let alone a mercury-related death, in this country from eating fish.

119

The widely heralded case at the Bay of Minimato in Japan where deaths occurred from mercury poisoning resulted from an unfortunate combination of circumstances: a plastics plant emptied mercury residue right into the bay; those who were affected ate an average of half a pound of the contaminated fish daily, and it is believed that some of them were workers in the plant where they also came into contact with the mercury. Levels of mercury in these fish bore no resemblance to levels present in the fish we consume. Mercury levels were 10 to 200 times higher, and these fish were consumed every day.

Mercury occurs in our environment naturally, in sea, soil, and food—all foods. It has probably always been in our environment. The important thing for us to do is to lessen and prevent increased pollution of the environment, not only with mercury but with other substances, too. There really are no safe or unsafe substances, only *safe or unsafe levels,* and safe and unsafe ways of using any substance. This requires a certain amount of common sense as well as scientific sense, and the two are not always the same!

Nations such as Sweden, Norway, Denmark, and Iceland, whose people eat many times the per capita amounts of fish that we do, have longevity and health records that equal or exceed ours. Our regulatory agencies should continue to monitor our foods for potentially harmful substances, but the application of common as well as scientific sense is necessary if we are to prevent further frustration of the consumer and of the food industry. Remember the cranberry fiasco of some years ago? What a bungle!

The best nutritional advice for the best of health is to have as varied a diet as possible—well balanced between the Basic Four Food Groups and the foods within these groups; and fish—including tuna and swordfish can and certainly should be included in the protein group.

The cautions that continue to be voiced relating to too many calories, too much saturated fat, cholesterol, and salt in the diet are the most important rules any consumer can follow. Your chances of becoming ill from mercury or other contaminants in the fish or other foods are infinitesimal compared with the hazards of too many calories and too much saturated fat and cholesterol.

Eat whatever variety of foods you like, eat them in moderation and enjoy them, for eating is one of the pleasures of life. Anything can be toxic if consumed in too large a quantity over too long a time. The mercury poisoning due to environmentally polluted fish from Minimato Bay is a glaring example of this. Here is another more recent illustration of a potential food hazard.

A RECIPE FOR SAFE FOOD: VARIETY AND COMMON SENSE

The Huckleby family from New Mexico provided some sensational ammunition for those who would sound the alarm on contaminated food on every hand. The journalists tended to focus far more on the fact that the Hucklebys were poisoned by pork containing mercury than on the errors in common sense and the rather unique aspects leading up to the poisoning. No doubt many readers read the publicity surrounding this episode and retained only the spine-chilling idea that pork can poison you because of the mercury it contains. The actual facts in the case were that the Huckleby family was poisoned by *repeatedly* eating pork from pigs that had been fed grain treated with mercury-containing fungicide and which was clearly marked *not* to be fed to animals. Surely this problem should never have developed if the caution had been heeded.

The key to safety in the food supply is heeding warnings such as that in the Huckleby's grain that they elected to feed to their pigs. The panic button response to potential hazards in food may lead large numbers of people to eliminate nutritionally important and actually safe foods from their usual diet pattern. Clearly, the numbers of persons who have suffered from nutritional deficiency diseases far outweigh even the obscure cases of poisoning resulting from eating without using common sense.

Analytical techniques for determining most substances have greatly improved in recent years, and it is possible now to detect tiny amounts of almost anything, where in the past this could not be done even though the substance in question was probably present. This is one important reason we can find DDT, mercury, lead, arsenic, and no doubt other potentially toxic substances if we look for them in practically anything—dill pickles, ice cream, organically fertilized foods, or a freshly washed knife, fork—even fingers.

It would probably have been more appropriate for the Food and Drug Administration to have restricted the use of foods and beverages containing cyclamates to people with diabetes. For persons with diabetes the tiny risk from cyclamates is far outweighed by the importance of restricting total calories in the diet.

But still there were many frightened cries about the contamination of food with mercury. This contaminant perhaps raised more interest in the food safety problem than any other single episode in recent years, although the banning of cyclamates obviously caused major financial adjustments in the food industry itself as well as unnecessary adjustments!

Hg—THE BUG-A-BOO METAL

Most of us think of mercury as the silvery material in the better quality thermometers or the difficult-to-pick-up metal we used in various high school chemistry experiments. When mercury is chemically combined with certain other substances, particularly if the resulting compound is soluble, as it is with mercury-containing fungicides and various salts used in the manufacture of certain chemicals, it can be absorbed in amounts that can be toxic.

Most recently it has been found that mercury salts, even inert mercury, can by the action of certain types of bacteria be converted into soluble, toxic organic compounds such as methyl and ethyl mercury.

Absorbable mercury—like lead, gold, and other heavy metals which are all naturally-occurring metals widely distributed in nature—tends to accumulate in certain body tissues such as bones, brain, and nerve tissues. A small amount even accumulates in muscle tissue. This is important because muscle tissue is the principal tissue we consume when we eat meat or fish. It doesn't take very much of an accumulation of mercury or other heavy metals to give rise to a variety of serious and usually irreversible physical problems. But the question is whether mercury contamination of our foods, not only fish but other foods, as well, *which we have always had,* has increased to a sufficiently high level to give cause for alarm. At present, it does not appear that this has happened, although we certainly must prevent it from doing so.

Despite the increasing amounts of tuna, swordfish, and other fish eaten in recent years, episodes of mercury poisoning other than the Hucklebys and the Minimato Bay cases have not been found. Fish is not the only food contaminated with mercury. For example, bread, potatoes, and meat may average about 0.1 part per million, and in the quantities they are consumed in our diets probably provide more mercury than fish having levels appreciably higher.

In March, 1970, the Food and Drug Administration quite arbitrarily decided that a general guideline of 0.5 parts per million of methyl mercury in fish is adequate to "protect the public." However, they also pointed out that "the 0.5 FDA guideline was not intended as a rigid rule." Thus, they left the possibility open that the 0.5 limit could be raised or lowered as new information became available. It is always better to err on the side of caution, and when the 0.5 ppm limit was first proposed, it might have been prudent. Now however, with more information available, with the realization that other more commonly consumed foods contribute more to our total mercury intake, the level of mercury permitted in fish has been increased to 1 ppm, as it is in Japan and one or two countries where consumption of fish is actually much higher than in the United States.

Certainly the FDA should continue to alert the public to potential hazards; they should increase monitoring our food supply not only for mercury, but also for other heavy metals, and they should encourage and support studies to learn more about the absorption, excretion, and tolerance of these and other potential contaminants in our environment. In the meantime and for the foreseeable future, it is safe to eat fish, including tuna and swordfish.

Remember, heart disease is the commonest cause of death in our society. Mercury poisoning from food is an extreme rarity. It has occurred only when the intake of mercury-contaminated food has been at an extremely high level and under most unusual circumstances. It would seem far more prudent to continue eating fish and more fish and take the very, very slight chance of mercury poisoning rather than the far greater chance of heart disease from (in part) an elevated level of cholesterol from (in part) an excessive consumption of saturated fats.

The Department of Chemical Engineering and Applied Chemistry of the University of Toronto, Canada, was one of the first to publish levels of mercury in several common foods. They found the lowest levels in eggs and the highest in dill pickles. Intermediate levels were reported in wheat, corn, rice, bread, milk, tea, several kinds of meats, vegetables, fruits, fish, and shellfish.

In determining our total mercury intake, it is important to consider not only the total mercury content of specific foods and the type of mercury compound present, but equally important, how often and in what quantities are the foods consumed? Dill pickles may contain 20 times the mercury of bread, but how many dill pickles does one eat compared with bread? Fish may have more mercury than beef or potatoes, but how often does one eat fish compared with beef and potatoes?

The really important problem of mercury contamination is to begin as soon as possible to prevent any further increase of mercury in our environment and to decrease the known sources of contamination. This is not the responsibility of our FDA except for whatever suggestions they can pass on to the appropriate federal and state agencies or legislation they may be helpful in initiating.

Even substances such as monosodium glutamate (MSG), which have been added to foods for years, now are being viewed with considerable suspicion and outright avoidance.

MSG—CYCLAMATE'S SUCCESSOR IN THE LIMELIGHT

MSG seems to have been re-labeled in some people's minds these days as Mighty Suspicious Goods (MSG). MSG has been widely used as a food flavor enhancer since the turn of this century. Products naturally rich in MSG had been used for centuries in food preparation to enhance flavor. In this country it is widely used by food processors to restore or enhance flavor lost in harvesting, preparation, and distribution. Housewives and chefs often sprinkle a little of it on many foods. The Chinese use it lavishly.

Scores of observations in the last quarter-century have demonstrated its safety for this purpose. Monosodium glutamate is a natural product which is converted to glutamic acid, a constituent of all protein foods, in the digestive process. Every day far more glutamic acid is obtained from the protein in our diets than may be added to foods as a flavor enhancer. Based on the extensive knowledge of MSG, the Food and Drug Administration has long carried MSG on its list of some 680 food substances "generally regarded as safe," or the well-known "GRAS" list.

The first criticism of MSG was something of a joke. The *New England Journal of Medicine* published a few letters reporting certain symptoms, including flushing and tightness in the face muscles, in some individuals after eating at Chinese restaurants. Two scientists said their experiments showed the cause to be MSG.

The editors of the *Journal* treated this as a great "put-on," referring to the symptoms as the "martini syndrome" and "Chinese temples," but the term "Chinese restaurant syndrome" finally stuck. However, the lay press took it seriously. The *Wall Street Journal* headlined it as a "mysterious malady."

A physician at the Department of Psychiatry of Washington University, St. Louis, published a report that he had found brain damage in newborn mice following injection of massive amounts of MSG under the skin. Similar observations were reported from the same investigator in a single infant monkey. To leap from these still independently unconfirmed experiments to the conclusion that MSG is harmful to babies in small amounts in some foods is hazardous, but many people—most of them laymen—have made the jump.

In doing so they created a wave of publicity that forced baby food producers to stop using MSG, even while protesting that years of use and experimentation had shown it to be safe. The potshots at MSG are unwarranted but unfortunately, they continue! Actually, MSG has been the subject of intensive laboratory investigations in the United States and Japan. Currently, several university and private laboratories are conducting research with this food flavor enhancer. While they continue exploring the safety of MSG, it may be of comfort to chefs and housewives to learn that the great bulk of scientific evidence favors the safety of MSG.

One review of the literature on MSG cites 29 references to scientific papers. With the exception of one study that reported the "Chinese restaurant syndrome" when large quantities of MSG were served to fasting human volunteers, and the previously reported study on the injection of MSG in newborn mice, the papers showed MSG was safe to both animals and man when used in a normal manner as a food flavor enhancer. Work in progress should determine definitively whether the preliminary alarms that have been raised are true or false.

The danger of prematurely publicizing scientific findings is that they can badly mislead and unnecessarily excite the public. For instance, a long-continued study at St. Louis University found that, under some circumstances, MSG in the diet can reduce blood cholesterol levels in man and certain animals. This is interesting, but inconclusive without a great deal more research. Nobody has made, nor should they make, any claims about MSG as a drug to reduce blood cholesterol. On the other hand, it is dangerous to make claims about MSG as a dangerous substance on the basis of tests where it was injected in very large amounts.

MSG is only one of the many additives used in foods. It is used to enhance flavor. The same reason is given for using saccharin or other sweeteners in various food products. However, these additives, like all others introduced into the food supply, must be approved by the Food and Drug Administration for use as an additive. Controversy has swirled around the approval process, as noted below.

DELANEY ET AL.!

After the banning of cyclamates as sweetening agents because of their supposed potential carcinogenic nature, attention turned intensely toward saccharin, the sweetener which was considered to have proven its safety by being used by diabetics and others over a period of many, many years with no ill effects manifesting themselves. The action on cyclamates was taken because this sweetener did not measure up to the stringent specifications of a clause in the Food Additives Amendment of 1958. This clause is called "The Delaney Clause," named after its author, Representative James J. Delaney of New York. The Delaney Clause is a part of a legislative package called the Food Additives Amendments of 1958. These amendments followed almost eight years of Congressional and public debate about the utility and safety of added chemicals in foods.

The original Congressional hearings on the issue of chemical food additives were held in 1951 under the chairmanship of Rep. Delaney of New York. Congressman Delaney believed that the Food and Drug Act of 1937 did not provide consumers with adequate safety protection against potentially harmful chemical additives because it did not require chemicals to be tested before they were marketed in foods. A similar provision for the pre-market testing of drugs had been included in the 1937 law, and the Congressman believed food safety demanded equally stringent controls.

In those and subsequent hearings in 1956, 1957, and 1958, a consensus developed among scientists, food manufacturers, and consumers that such a testing requirement was indeed necessary, but there was substantial disagreement about which substances should be examined. Everyone realized that vast numbers of chemicals were already widely used in foods, and to require the Food and Drug Administration or the food processors to test each one adequately would far outstrip available scientific resources. Neither was everyone agreed on the need to test chemicals exclusively for cancer or any other single disease.

On this point, the FDA was particularly concerned. In an opinion written in 1958, the agency noted, "We, of course, agree that no chemical should be permitted to be used in food if, as so used, it may cause cancer. No specific reference to carcinogens is necessary for this purpose, however, since the general requirements of this bill give assurance that no chemical additive can be cleared if there is a reasonable doubt about its safety in that respect."

Many Congressmen agreed with this position and didn't see any particular need for including the anti-cancer clause in the amendments. For that reason, the clause was not included in the bill when it was presented on the House floor for debate. However, Congressman Delaney strongly believed that this was an essential part of the food safety package, and following some behind-the-scenes persuasion, the anti-cancer clause was reinserted into the amendments after the debate had ended. The House voted to pass the complete amendments intact rather than prolong arguments over the need to single out cancer for special attention.

The Senate followed the House lead and passed the amendments with no modifications. However, the Senate report on the bill noted that, "We want the record to show that in our opinion the bill is aimed at preventing the addition to the food our people eat of any substance, the ingestion of which reasonable people would expect to produce not just cancer, but any disease or disability. In short, we believe the bill reads the same with or without the inclusion of the clause referred to."

Curiously, when the anti-cancer clause was again proposed for inclusion in the Color Additive Amendments of 1960, the FDA made a complete about face in its view of the Delaney Clause. Whereas the agency had originally regarded the clause as an irrelevant, but harmless rider on the food additives amendments, it now believed it was an absolutely essential component of the color additives legislation.

In part, this change in attitude was the result of a change in administration following President Kennedy's succession of President Eisenhower. However, it was also a highly conservative response to a National Cancer Institute report on cancer-causing agents. This report concluded, "No one at this time can tell how much or how little of a carcinogen would be required to produce a cancer in any human being, or how long it would take the cancer to develop." The agency thus reaffirmed the absolute approach of the Delaney Clause to food safety on the basis of this uncertainty.

But this concept of zero cancer risk does not apply consistently across the board. The authority of the Delaney Clause is limited strictly to those chemicals which are labeled as food additives. The clause does not have the authority to ban naturally-occurring carcinogens, such as aflatoxins or black pepper, those chemicals approved before 1958, such as nitrites, or accidental environmental contaminants, such as PCBs.

The National Academy of Sciences has suggested that our food laws need revising to permit more flexibility. One aspect of the law which the NAS committee studying the problem identified as "inflexible" is the Delaney Clause. The Delaney Clause strictly forbids the use of a chemical in any amount in foods if it has been found by appropriate tests to cause cancer in man or animals. While this approach is basically sound, the all-or-nothing attitude that the Clause exemplifies is too rigid in light of today's knowledge about cancer to be effective as a regulatory policy.

In the past few years, we have learned that our food supply contains a wide variety of potentially carcinogenic substances, both natural and man-made. These chemicals differ substantially in their toxic potency, yet most are found in foods in very minute concentrations. Aflatoxins, for example, have been described as the most potent liver carcinogens known, but are found in peanuts and some grain products in only a few parts per billion. In contrast, saccharin, with its cancer-causing activity still the subject of controversy, is estimated to be more than a million times less potent than aflatoxins—if it causes human cancer at all. Yet aflatoxins are permitted in foods at certain restricted levels, while the FDA has taken regulatory steps against saccharin.

Because of this inconsistency, the NAS report advised that our food laws be modified so that we might be able to classify possible cancer-causing chemicals according to their degree of risk. This, of course, would mean that the absolute prohibition demanded by the Delaney Clause would also have to be modified.

In its place, the NAS panel suggested a law that would allow a number of regulatory alternatives to be applied, depending on the severity of the risk, the special needs of particular consumers, or the benefits that might offset a small cancer risk. Under its proposed new system, potential cancer risks would be classified by some rough scheme, such as high, medium, or low. This classification, in turn, would direct the FDA to one or more possible actions. For high cancer risks, there is little doubt that a total ban on food uses would be the most effective means of ensuring safety. For medium or low cancer risks, a complete ban may be inappropriate.

Depending on the particular nature of the cancer risk and the intended use of the substance in foods, it might be more effective to limit use or availability to a special segment of the population, in the same way that we now discourage children from buying cigarettes or liquor.

In other circumstances, it might be possible to allow the use of a potentially carcinogenic substance, but at levels below those originally proposed. A useful additive in some processing method, for example, might be used at three parts per million rather than at 10 or 20 parts per million.

Low-risk foods or ingredients may not warrant anything more than a warning label or logo that would advise consumers of a possible—but remote—chance of illness. Such a warning perhaps could discourage certain consumers, such as pregnant women, not to consume a certain food product during pregnancy when a potential hazard might be more serious. Or a label might suggest that overconsumption of a specific food should be avoided.

The underlying premise of these proposed changes is that the regulatory process should include more responsibility for individual consumers rather than the more authoritarian system operating now. This, of course, also assumes that most consumers will be able to modify their own personal behaviors after learning about food hazards. Such assumptions are certainly subject to controversy.

American eaters are uneasy and have remained nervous about their food ever since the banning of cyclamates some 12 years ago. Since then, they have been told in a barrage of books and articles that the chemicals in food are lurking in the pantry, just waiting for the opportunity to pollute their systems and scramble the genes of the next generation! Fear of cancer, widespread and understandable, plus the inconsistencies and inflexibility of our food regulatory system seem to be responsible for the continuing panic-in-the-pantry phenomenon and the associated rush to "health foods."

Cancer, in its many forms, is one of the most prevalent and least understood of all diseases. Its incidence, in part because of longer life expectancy, has increased since 1900; it is now second only to heart disease as a cause of death in the United States. Because we don't fully understand the origin of cancer, we tend to suspect just about everything in our environment. This certainly applies to additives in the food supply. Yet the increase in cancer is primarily due to a marked increase in cancer of the lungs related to smoking.

Our food legislation today promotes hasty, irrational bannings of perfectly safe and useful food additives. The so-called "Delaney Anti-cancer Clause," part of the 1958 Food Additives Amendment, states that any additive that is found to induce cancer when ingested by man or animal must be removed from the market. At first glance, the Delaney Clause might sound reasonable. Obviously, none of us would want to eat a food if it causes cancer. However, food chemicals are being banned at the drop of a rat, and consumer anxieties are mounting without cause, because of the mere existence of this legislation. Whether or not the clause is formally invoked, it has created a situation where any additive can be banned without any supportive evidence.

The inflexibility and inconsistencies of the Delaney Clause bring up several critical questions which are particularly relevant as saccharin undergoes review. First, the rigidity of the regulation leaves no room for scientific discretion. Thus one animal experiment, regardless of the dosage used, which reveals cancer may result in a banning of that additive. Shouldn't we have, instead, a series of experiments by a variety of scientists, using various dosages, before action is taken?

Second, the lack of flexibility of the Delaney Clause presents serious problems. For example, an additive (like nitrite) performs a unique, health-promoting function (the prevention of botulism), but is linked with animal cancer in one or two high-dose experiments, so its future is in doubt. Shouldn't the consequences of its withdrawal from foods be taken into account before action is taken?

Third, to apply those rigid rules to artificial additives and not to natural foods is inconsistent. An overdose of vitamin A brings about cancer in rats (and is highly toxic to humans), but vitamin A is not banned. Why should one chemical be banned because it is artificial and another exonerated because it is natural? Shouldn't we be concerned in a rational, scientific way about the safety of all foods, no matter what their origin?

Fourth, another look at the relevance of animal overdosing experiments is imperative. How can you make generalizations to human beings from feeding rodents amounts of cyclamates equal to over one thousand bottles of diet soda a day?

Fifth, cancer can develop in some animal species or strains when exposed to a chemical, but not in others. How can we be guided by the results which could be explained by the sensitivity of one particular type of animal?

In spite of all its shortcomings, the Delaney Clause is still in effect and ruling our land. Consequently, considerable press attention is given to self-appointed consumer advocates who make a career out of calling attention to isolated animal experiments, usually involving astronomical dosages over long periods, that link food additives with cancer. The consumer sees the word "cancer" in the headlines, anxiety mounts, and the 100 percent natural life looks appealing.

The current flight from chemicals is a double-barreled source of concern. It can cause a loss of the immediate health benefits offered by additives, and the fascination with no-artificial-anything menus may mask the real health threats, such as cigarette smoking, lack of exercise, and just plain overeating. Also, the omission of additives and an interruption in food chemical research, in our ongoing effort to improve food availability and quality, can only result in one large nutritional step—backward.

SWEET TALK

Although discussions about saccharin often focus on the possible carcinogenicity of this sweetener, there are some arguments in favor of using this product. A government report on the benefits of saccharin identified several groups who conceivably benefit from saccharin availability. They are: diabetics; the obese and those concerned with weight control; individuals susceptible to tooth decay; persons with special dietary restrictions; and those who must take certain types of medication.

For most of these groups, saccharin is beneficial as a sugar substitute. In the U.S., where there is a heavy cultural emphasis on sweet foods, enormous psychological pressure is exerted on those who must strictly control their intake of sugar. Because it is calorie-free, saccharin offers these individuals a chance to enjoy the sweet taste of many foods without the hazards that might result from sugar's calories.

Diabetes—For diabetics, strict control of total caloric intake and a decrease in the amount of sugar consumed is essential to health. Many diabetics, who may number more than 10 million in the U.S., believe the availability of saccharin helps them to maintain their restrictive diets and at the same time eat many kinds of sweet foods. Although saccharin is not essential to the maintenance of a diabetic's health, many physicians agree that it makes their patients' lives a bit more enjoyable.

Obesity—It has been estimated that more than 50 million Americans suffer from obesity, and many more are seriously concerned with weight control. The essence of weight reduction is decreased caloric intake, or "negative energy balance." Simply, this means that to lose weight, a person must ingest fewer calories than needed in order to use up energy stored as excess fat.

Many Americans believe saccharin is beneficial to their efforts to lose or control weight. Dieters think it helps them avoid sugar and stay on their diets. There is little evidence, however, that using saccharin does, in fact, lead people to lose weight, or once lost, to maintain a lower body weight.

Another less well-defined group includes persons who are not seriously concerned with obesity, but use saccharin to help them stay at a preferred weight level. These individuals, despite the absence of a valid medical reason, like saccharin because of the freedom it allows in meal planning. For instance, someone might prefer a diet soda at lunchtime in order to have an extra glass of wine or cocktail with dinner and still balance total caloric intake. And although no scientific evidence is available on these persons, the surprisingly negative consumer reaction to the proposed saccharin ban probably included many with these convictions.

Dental caries—Sugar, because it is a carbohydrate, contributes to dental caries (tooth decay), which affects virtually everyone. As a sugar substitute, it is reasonable to think that saccharin could be beneficial by reducing exposure to sugar and thus reducing the incidence of dental caries. No studies of these possible benefits have been conducted. Saccharin's sweet taste is also supposed to encourage good oral hygiene practices like regular brushing, particularly among children. Almost every brand of toothpaste contains saccharin as a flavoring additive.

Saccharin is a popular sweetener, but there are a couple of other sweeteners now available for those consumers who are concerned about saccharin as an additive. Aspartame is an amino acid-based sweetener consisting of a molecule of aspartic acid and one of phenylalanine. This is a very sweet substance which can be used in small amounts for sweetening various foods. The other interesting new sweetener is fructose. Fructose, a simple sugar, has been known a long time, but it was not available in the market because of its high cost. The price is still high, but some consumers are interested in using it because it is a far more effective sweetener in water than is sucrose. However, baked products require table sugar (sucrose) and fructose in approximately comparable amounts. Consequently, fructose affords essentially no saving in calories in baked products.

Those of us who specialize in nutrition are pleased by the great public interest in the relationship between food and health. We are pleased because a knowledge of nutrition is essential to homemakers, chefs, administrators in institutions responsible for feeding people, and in fact, is essential to all of us to prevent malnutrition in this land of plenty.

However, we also get upset by the misinformation, half-facts, and conclusion-jumping that appear in the media to mislead or even frighten the public. To educate the public in scientific findings is one thing, to expose the public to inconclusive test results without explaining them is quite another. In still another realm of our food supply, comment has often been far more emotional than rational.

AGRICULTURAL CHEMICALS

The current hysteria about agricultural chemicals has seeped in under the doorsills of American homes all across the land.

One woman said recently, "I feel like Lucretia Borgia every time I put dinner on the table. Am I poisoning my family?"

That concerned woman, interested primarily in the health and well-being of her family, deserves to have an end put to her confusion about agricultural chemicals, particularly pesticides. Her bafflement stems not from stupidity, but from the claims and counter-claims of self-appointed experts who all too frequently are ill-informed themselves. They are usually extrapolating to man some findings on birds, bees, or fish, or the unfortunate result of some child inhaling or swallowing large quantities of some pesticide. Such matters just don't extend to the use of agricultural chemicals in the growing, protecting, or preserving of foods.

Let's set aside all arguments about how or why the current controversy started and concentrate instead on letting facts speak for themselves.

One irrefutable fact is this simple statement: *There is not one medically documented instance of ill health in man, not to mention death, that can be attributed to the proper use of pesticides, or even to their improper use as far as ill health from residues on foods.* If anyone can bring forward any evidence to refute this statement, there are many agencies such as the Food and Drug Administration, the Public Health Service, and the Food Protection Committee of the Food and Nutrition Board that would welcome an opportunity to investigate the case.

In spite of this lack of evidence, many people have the impression that pesticides contaminate our food supply, are harmful, and probably lethal. This gap between fact and fancy must be closed or we will do ourselves great harm by allowing disease and famine to rule the earth.

Are pesticides poison? Of course they are. That's why they work. They are poison to the insects, worms, rats, weeds and other living pests against which they are designed to be directed. Because of strictly enforced regulations and tolerance levels, however, the hazard to man from pesticide residues on foods is very, very small. Pesticides are dangerous if you handle them carelessly or leave them around where children may drink them or play with them.

You can have confidence in our foods. They are not full of poisons, but are full of important nutrients, and the quality is much better for eating pleasure than it was a generation ago. Eat and enjoy them.

A committee of the Food and Nutrition Board of the National Academy of Science issued this statement on insecticides: "We could not have arrived at the position of power we now hold as a nation had we not made our agriculture so efficient."

WHY PESTICIDES?

As one expert expressed it, "The only hope, if we are to feed and clothe a growing population, is to control the pests." Experts feel that chemicals must be used if the food and health of the nation are to be maintained. First of all, it is essential to realize that even our present crop production will not be enough to meet the demands of our exploding world population. More and more people mean not only more mouths to feed, but also more land used for homes and industry and less and less land for farms. Yet total yield must increase.

This means increasing the amount of food one acre will produce. It also means decreasing the huge and needless losses by insects, fungi, bacteria, viruses, and weeds. They are able to destroy an average of one-fifth of the total crop every year.

For instance, potatoes are subject to attack by at least 200 insects and disease agents. In the nine years after organic pesticides were introduced, the average yield of potatoes per acre was increased by 90 per cent. Furthermore, use of pesticides to eliminate flies (including the Mediterranean fruit fly), mosquitoes, and intestinal parasites has improved pork and beef production and increased milk output.

It is recognized, of course, that proper controls must be vigilantly applied. Nonchemical ways of insect control are being used as much as possible and much research has been directed toward new means such as interference with reproduction to help control insect populations. The Food and Drug Administration is concentrating on methods for measuring residues in foods so that now even miniscule amounts of insecticides can be determined. The U.S. Public Health Service is studying how to decrease water pollution, how to improve control of aerial application of pesticides, and how to educate farmers and the public against carelessness in the use of pesticides.

Food processors, too, are making a contribution. They have carefully trained field men to supervise growers, to oversee application of pesticides, and to insure the elapse of an appropriate amount of time between application and harvest. In the field and at the processing plant, samples are analyzed so that residues are below the tolerance levels both before and after processing. It is clear that controls need to be improved and a watchdog diligence must be maintained, but *pesticides are and will continue to be safe with appropriate supervision and regulation.*

Perhaps pesticides and automobiles should be compared. They both are a source of accidents and worry, and the need for protection against them is great. Nevertheless, they cannot be abolished without losing tremendous benefits. Pesticides properly used are essential to provide good nutrition today and to prevent starvation in the future.

SOME COMMON SENSE COMMENTS ON PESTICIDES AND FERTILIZERS

Much of the consumer's concern about pesticides stems from a worry over how much of the pesticide remains on the food when it reaches the table. Many people have asked about the best way to wash pesticide residues from fresh produce.

If you've ever visited a commercial cannery or frozen food factory and watched the gallons and gallons of water used to wash the food that is to be processed, you soon became aware of the merits of just plain water in preparing food. And with fresh fruits and vegetables in the home, it is up to you to use a little common sense and the kitchen sink. The Food and Drug Administration writes that fresh fruits and vegetables should be washed thoroughly in clean water. This, however, would not assure the removal of pesticides in all cases because some of the residues are not soluble in water and some are translocated by being introduced into the root system directly into the food rather than being concentrated on the surface.

It is possible that some detergents would be helpful in washing fruits and vegetables, but the particular detergent would have to be carefully selected and the food rinsed very well to avoid the possibility of objectionable residues from the detergent itself. However, clean water is the right choice for removing much of the very small amount of residue that may remain on the produce. In most cases, the residues on the unwashed food are within the safe legal tolerances established under the Federal Food, Drug, and Cosmetic Act. Even without washing well, there is no evidence of sickness in man from consuming pesticide residues on foods.

From time to time concern is voiced not so much about the effects of today's pesticides, but more in relation to the pesticides of the future. It is not unusual to hear that insects may develop resistance to some of the insecticides currently in use. The logical sequence to that development could be a more powerful insecticide, followed by acquired resistance, development of a still more powerful insecticide, and on and on, ad infinitum. The logic breaks down, however, when one assumes that the new insecticide must be more powerful. So far it has been possible to shift to other, not necessarily stronger insecticides to overcome the problem. Of course, new insecticides will need to be tested carefully to insure that residues are not left at levels that even remotely could harm humans.

Another hotly contested point is the use of commercial fertilizers rather than growing foods in soil that is termed "organic." The use of fertilizers has long been proven as an effective means of increasing crop yields. Some land that has been farmed for very brief periods of time contains sufficient nutrients for plants to flourish, but much of today's farm land has been tilled for crop after crop after crop. Not surprisingly, this has caused a depletion of some of the nutrients in the soil that plants need for optimum growth. This situation is analogous to the need of humans for adequate amounts of essential nutrients if optimum growth and health are to be achieved. The addition of fertilizer to a crop is simply a practical way of insuring the food that plants need to produce our food. The fertilizer, whether organic or chemical, does not alter the protein, carbohydrate, fat, or vitamin content of the food on a pound per pound comparison with the same plant grown without fertilizer. However, the total amount of food produced on an acre, hence the total amount of protein, carbohydrate, fat, and vitamins available from this acre, is *significantly increased* when the correct nutrients are supplied with fertilizer. Fertilizers may very slightly influence the mineral content of the food raised if soluble minerals such as iodine are included in the fertilizer. However, the chief factor in determining nutritive value of a serving of food raised is the genetic qualities of the *seed* used.

Before winding up this chapter, let's take a brief look at some of the factors that are important in procuring healthful shellfish.

THESE "R" THE DAYS!

With the emphasis on back to nature and enjoying the increasing leisure available to many Americans, maybe a reminder on shellfish is due.

No doubt you are familiar with the adage that oysters should be eaten only in months with an R in their names. This would mean that January, February, March, April, September, October, November, and December are all good months for eating oysters, but stay away from oysters in May, June, July, and August! Apparently this axiom originated when it was observed that oysters eaten in the summer months sometimes caused people to become ill. We now know that other shellfish such as clams and mussels also can cause this shellfish poisoning during these months. Shellfish poisoning is caused when you eat any shellfish that has been eating a one-celled organism called *Gonyaulax catanella*. This organism is a popular food for shellfish and flourishes in coastal waters during the warm summer months, sometimes concentrating in such large numbers that they cause an unusual fluorescence in the ocean water. At night you can see the fluorescent glow from the water, and in the daytime you can notice a distinctly reddish color, which accounts for the common name "Red Tide." These signs are positive proof that the *Gonyaulax catanella* concentration is very high. However, shellfish are dangerous to eat when they are removed from waters with even a much lower concentration of this organism. The surprising thing is that this organism doesn't seem to harm the shellfish even at very high concentrations, but the poison from the organism concentrated in the shellfish causes shellfish poisoning when eaten by humans.

The poison will dissipate from oysters fairly quickly when they are held in fresh water. It disappears more slowly from mussels, and butter clams give up the poison very slowly when held in clear water. Possible hazard from shellfish during the summer months can be somewhat reduced by holding the shellfish in clear water for a while. Danger is further reduced by frying the shellfish in oil and eating them as part of a large meal rather than as a snack by themselves. These precautions should certainly be observed if you insist on clamming on your own during the summer months.

Most of us get shellfish from commercial sources rather than by making our own jaunt to the beach. Clams and mussels are harvested under government control. Chemical tests are run to detect even extremely small amounts of the poison. Commercial canneries greatly reduce the amount of poison that might possibly be present at the beginning of processing by using live steam to remove the poison. Certainly it is wise to be aware of the possibility of shellfish poisoning, because it can be fatal within two hours after the poisoned shellfish is eaten. However, you can be confident that commercially processed shellfish are safe.

If you happen to be an ardent clamdigger, just heed the old adage about eating shellfish only in months with an R in their names.

No doubt other concerns will crop up to alarm the public about the safety of our food supply. Vigilance is always important so that adequate standards will be maintained at all times. However, panic can trigger inappropriate and possibly harmful action. An inquiring, but not an emotional attitude will be a real asset in the increasingly complex world as innovations are developed to meet the need for more and more food.

6

FOOD MANAGEMENT TIPS

Cleanliness and purity in our food are taken for granted by most people in this country. We are so accustomed to inspection marks and sterilized containers that we are apt to forget how much care this involves. Actually, for the food to be absolutely safe at the time it is eaten good sanitation must be assured from the time of harvest or slaughter until the food is consumed. With today's specialized world and urbanization, a safe food supply requires appropriate legislation, technically competent food processors, enforcement agencies, conscientious food merchandisers, and an educated consumer.

Government legislation has established appropriate standards of sanitation and the means necessary for enforcing the legislation. States are responsible for establishing and maintaining standards on food raised and consumed within one state, and the federal government regulates all food that crosses state lines. Food processors have conducted extensive research to insure that the food is handled in the plant so that it is safe to pass through the normal marketing chain. These manufacturers have taken the initiative in developing such conveniences for the consumer as a "tin" can which can safely be used for storing leftovers in their own cans in the refrigerator. These aspects of the food supply have been closely supervised.

The safety of food once it reaches the hands of the consumer is a matter of individual responsibility. Persons preparing food in the home will be able to maintain a safe standard of sanitation if a few fundamental ideas are kept in mind.

Here are a few tips about handling food. Remember that food handled outside of its original wrapping has been exposed to increased contamination even when you have been very careful. The bacteria present in food multiply very rapidly at room temperature, and grow more readily in some types of food than in others. You can minimize food contamination by forming the habit of always

137

washing your hands thoroughly with soap and rinsing well before handling food. Be careful to keep your hands away from your mouth and nose and out of your hair when you are working with food. If you happen to sneeze or cough, move away from the food and cover your face with a handkerchief so the germs are not broadcast to the food. Be sure to wash your hands before returning to food preparation. Be careful to work with food only on clean areas and with clean utensils. Avoid leaving food such as milk, eggs, and meats at room temperature.

The subject of food safety is one that most of us prefer not to think about, but food poisoning does happen mostly as a result of improper storage or handling of food *in the home*. Since food safety can be insured with some knowledge and care in the kitchen, it seems wise to talk about this important, but somewhat unpleasant subject.

When you hear someone complaining about an upset stomach, the frequent comment is that it was just caused by something he ate. The truth is likely to be that the intestinal upset was actually a case of staphylococcus poisoning. Much of the hazard in foods has been reduced because fresh foods are generally handled quickly and kept under adequate refrigeration during the marketing process so that food is wholesome when it gets to you. From then on, the safety of the food is up to you. Research has shown that most microorganisms flourish at moderate temperatures. If you keep this fact in mind when handling food, you will always be careful to keep perishable food items either adequately refrigerated or in an oven heated above 140°F.

This means that it is important to take groceries home right after purchasing them without letting them sit in a hot car while you run several errands along the way. As soon as you get home, quickly put all perishable foods in the refrigerator or freezer. Foods that are particularly susceptible are meats, poultry, fish of all types, milk and other dairy items. Of course, all frozen foods should be put in the freezer before they can begin to thaw very much.

Your refrigerator should maintain a temperature between 33 and 40°F. The importance of storing perishable foods at temperatures just above freezing was demonstrated when a friend wrote that she had been sick off and on for several weeks and even been hospitalized with a mysterious ailment; it was finally shown to be caused by staphylococcal food poisoning resulting from storing food just above the safe storage temperature. It was finally found that her brand new refrigerator was holding foods between 45 and 50°F, a temperature at which the staph microorganisms could multiply, particularly in the milk.

To keep microbiological contamination of food to an absolute minimum, remove food from the refrigerator just before you begin to cook it. Avoid letting meats stand in an oven for several hours before the oven is programmed to begin heating the food. Most meats that are strictly fresh can be left two hours in a cold oven, but it is definitely unwise to put a roast in the oven before leaving for work in the morning and program the oven to turn on in the middle of the afternoon. However, frozen meat cuts can be used in this way because they will stay colder than 40 degrees for a long time as they thaw. Needless to say, gas ovens are warmer than electric ovens because of the pilot light, and therefore should have meats held in them for shorter periods before programming the roasting to begin.

You should also be careful to refrigerate leftovers very soon after a meal. It is not safe, for example, to leave a roast turkey filled with dressing on the kitchen counter for several hours. For maximum safety, strip the meat from the carcass and spoon out the leftover dressing and store in the refrigerator right after the meal.

Remember the foods that are most likely to spoil and cause food poisoning are meats, milk and egg-containing foods such as creamed dishes, salads such as chicken or tuna, and cream pies. Fresh fruits and vegetables need not be refrigerated as carefully since they are a poor medium for the growth of staph and other food-borne microorganisms that cause digestive upsets.

As you might guess from all this, picnics present difficulties in good food handling practices. However, they certainly need not end in a round of illness due to food poisoning.

HOT WEATHER HAZARDS

If you are planning menus for summer picnics, we hope you will plan for safety as well as for pleasure. What is true of fireworks and highways, or swimming and sunning, is also true of food. It can be hazardous as well as fun. And what applies to Memorial Day and July Fourth applies to all meals all summer long.

In the warm weather relaxing is fine, but definitely a poor plan when it comes to food. If you are careless in the kitchen, out in the yard, or on a picnic, you may a'l too quickly end up with an unexpected and most unpleasant case of food poisoning. Even mild cases cause hours or days of great intestinal misery, and severe cases may even cause death. Why is this a more common problem in the summer than in the rest of the year? Because the bacteria that are responsible for food poisoning grow rapidly in warm temperatures. All during the year these bacteria may be around the house, on pots and pans, on dishes and in dust, in and on people. Yet they do no damage when steaming food is eaten soon after it leaves the range, or when chilled food is served promptly after it is taken from the refrigerator. The difficulty comes in summer when food is left cooling or warming in hot kitchens and cars, on beaches, or out in the country. This is just what bacteria love. If even a few are present, they need only a few hours to change safe food into dangerous food. Even though the food may look and taste and smell as good as ever, it can make trouble for anyone who eats it.

The only way to prevent this is to prevent the conditions that encourage bacterial growth. Fortunately, with only a few precautions you can make sure that you will be safe and not sorry.

First of all, when you buy good clean foods, keep them that way. Our food supply is probably the safest in the world, but that does not mean we can treat it carelessly. During storage, food has to be put in spick and span containers, and if it needs to be kept cold, it should be refrigerated promptly. During preparation, it has to be protected, too. It cannot stay safe if it comes in contact with dirty hands, with a sore on the skin, or with droplets from a sneeze or cough.

Finally, prepared food must also be handled with care. If cooked food which is to be eaten later is at home, it should be cooled and refrigerated fast. If it is going on a picnic, it should be put in containers which will keep it boiling hot for all the hours between heating time and eating time. Chilled food must be kept icy cold. It should never, but never, warm up. Many of the hazards of picnics can be removed thanks to those handy portable ice chests. You can pack potato salad and meats of your choice in these chests to keep cold until you plan to eat.

Be particularly careful with milk, eggs, meat, fish, poultry, and all the mixtures that contain them. Be equally cautious with salad combinations, and pies and pastries. If you can't pack them properly, plan a different menu, one that relies on foods in cans that may be opened at the last minute and foods that can be grilled on the spot.

The more common food poisoning problems due to poor sanitation and improper storage practices that we have just been describing are chiefly caused by *Staphylococci, Salmonellae,* and *Streptococci.* "Staph" causes food poisoning by producing a toxin as it multiplies; the other two largely by the presence of very large numbers of bacteria rather than any toxin produced.

There is also a highly toxic food poisoning known as botulism.

PRECAUTIONS ON HOME-CANNED VEGETABLES

Botulism, fortunately, is a fairly rare problem in the United States, so rare that cases usually end up in the newspaper nationwide. *Clostridium botulinum* thrives in the absence of air. As it grows, this bacterium produces a powerful and deadly toxin, rated to be more deadly than venom from the cobra! As little as 0.01 milligrams of the *Cl. botulinum* toxin can be fatal. In fact, in one episode improperly processed ripe olives contained enough toxin that one olive was sufficient to cause death.

The organism may be dormant or inactive as a spore, and in this form may be found in the intestinal tract of animals and in soil. If this spore contaminates food which isn't properly processed, and the food is stored in a warm, tight container with no access to air, the spore begins to grow and produce the toxin.

Botulism also differs from the common types of food poisoning in that the usual warning and protective symptoms of diarrhea, nausea, or vomiting do not appear in the customary three to six hours after eating the contaminated food. Instead, after eating a product contaminated with the toxin of botulism, neurological symptoms such as muscular weakness, headache, paralysis of the muscles involved in swallowing, moving the eyes, and in breathing will develop. These may appear within a few hours, usually within 24 hours, but may be delayed for from two to six days. Death results from heart or breathing paralysis.

The spore itself is quite heat resistant, but the toxin is readily destroyed by boiling. A temperature of 248°F must be maintained for at least ten minutes in order to kill the spore. Obviously, this elevated temperature can only be reached in a pressure cooker. The toxin, however, is inactivated simply by boiling the food containing the poison for fifteen to twenty minutes, a measure which can be handled with ordinary equipment. .

Most cases of botulism in the United States, but not all, have been due to improper home canning and insufficient heating before eating vegetables and meat or fish products. Corn, beans, spinach, and mushrooms are particularly famous (or infamous) as home-canned carriers of the toxin. Fruits present less of a hazard because of their distinctly more acidic medium, which is less favorable to the growth of the bacteria.

All home canned vegetables, meats, or other protein food should be thoroughly heated (boiled for 20 minutes) before tasting. Commercial canning of food is now carried out on such a scientific basis that there is usually less danger of botulism from this source. However, there may always be the rare exception. Beware of any bulging cans, cans from which gas escapes when opened, or any food with an "off" odor or color. The bulging of the cans is a sign that the bacteria have been growing, and when the bacteria grow they produce the toxin along with the gas.

Antitoxins have been developed that are vital in treatment, but the particular type of organism causing botulism must be identified before treatment with the proper antitoxin can be initiated. A 20-minute boiling period before serving home-canned vegetables and meats is an effective means of preventing the problem, and this is clearly a thousand times better than the treatment.

TRICHINOSIS CAN BE FEROCIOUS

Although this title may be somewhat "à la Ogden Nash," it points up another aspect of food preparation that is simple to manage if the cook is merely informed of a general rule about cooking pork. Occasionally pigs are fed untreated garbage and this may cause the pigs to harbor a parasite known as trichinae. These trichinae may in turn be part of a pork cut when the pig is sold as pork in the consumer market. The trichinae are still viable even though the host is not. Therefore, some measure must be taken to insure that the trichinae are killed before the meat is eaten. The dead trichinae may not be pleasant to think about, but they present no hazard to the diner. However, if viable trichinae are eaten, the hapless diner becomes the new host and he develops trichinosis, a parasitic disease which tends to drain one's strength and energy, but which is not fatal.

To put this into perspective, pigs that are fed garbage these days generally are given garbage that has been treated to make the presence of trichinae impossible. However, there is still a remote chance that pork may contain this parasite; so a word of caution seems advisable.

Freezing and cooking are two common ways available to the consumer to destroy trichinae. Fresh pork must always be heated to a minimum temperature of 137°F in all parts in order to kill the organism. Actually, it is wise to exceed this temperature significantly just to build in a margin of safety since the meat cut will not be a uniform temperature throughout. General practice has been to heat pork to 185°F interior temperature, although a temperature of 170°F has not only proven perfectly safe, but also very palatable. If you don't have a meat thermometer to check the temperature, you can use the color of the interior of the muscle as a guide. Pork (uncured) will change to a gray color, losing all trace of pink, by the time the meat reaches 170°F. If even a trace of pink is showing, you would be wise to cook the meat a little longer.

Freezing temperatures must be maintained at a maximum temperature of 5°F or cooler for at least 12 days for very thin cuts to as long as 30 days for thick cuts of pork. It is recommended that the frozen storage temperature be maintained in the range of −10°F to −20°F so that the organism will be killed more quickly.

One common means of preparing pork for the market is to smoke it. Smokehouse temperatures vary from 109 to 159°F. If pork is hung for an extended period at the higher temperature, the trichinae will be killed, but not at lower temperatures. Since the consumer is not present when the manufacturer is smoking the bacon or ham he may ultimately buy, one has to cook these smoked products at home to insure that the meat reaches a high enough temperature to kill the trichinae that might be (but rarely are) present.

As a matter of interest, meats are cured or smoked for several reasons: to aid in preservation, to give distinctive flavors to foods, and to impart a desirable appearance. The ingredients permitted in curing bacon bearing the marks of inspection of the Meat Inspection Division of the U.S. Department of Agriculture are: sodium chloride (salt), sugar, sodium nitrate, sodium nitrite, and vinegar. There are four general types of curing: dry cure, pickle cure, injection cure, and the method used in finely ground products like sausage meat in which the cure is mixed into the product. Some products are further treated by smoking. All pork products prepared in federally inspected establishments that might be used in the home without thorough cooking (including smoked hams, smoked sausages, etc.) are required to be treated by one of the recognized methods for the destruction of trichinae before release from the processing establishment.

A good motto of health is: Always cook your bacon—and why not cook it crisp to get rid of much of the fat?

After reading the various warnings in this chapter, you probably agree with us that good health can only be achieved from good food properly handled. Although this book is basically planned to help in learning to eat the foods required for good health, we included the information needed to keep those good foods in good condition for you to eat safely.

Even when menus are planned carefully, there are still many decisions to be made in the supermarket or grocery store, decisions that can make a good bit of difference in the price tag attached to your basket of groceries and in the nutrients in those foods you've picked.

LABELS—YOUR GUIDE TO NUTRITION AND ECONOMY

Smart shoppers today need to read labels on many food items in the grocery store, even if it means getting out the bifocals to read the fine print! There is a lot of information on a label if you will just take the time to read it. For economy's sake, it is wise to read the amount contained in a package so that you can compare the cost per ounce of one brand with that of another brand. Such a comparison helps your pocketbook, but it requires more attention to the label to be sure about the nutrition you are buying in various brands.

Federal law requires that a label must list all the ingredients in a product, and that these ingredients must be listed in order of the amount contained in the product. The first ingredient listed on a label is the item contained in the largest amount. The second ingredient listed is present in a smaller amount than the first ingredient, and so on. This information is very helpful when you compare different brands of a particular product. For instance, a meat soup in which the meat is listed close to the beginning of the list of ingredients would contain more meat than a comparable soup in which the meat is one of the last ingredients listed.

As you go through the grocery store, you will find many foods labeled with a long list of ingredients, but others that list no ingredients at all. This may sound like the government is being very fussy about some food products and completely ignoring others. Thus mayonnaise does not have a list of ingredients on its label, but most salad dressings do. The reason for this is that standards of identity have been carefully spelled out, and it is legally permissible to market these standardized products with just a label naming the product. Of course, the manufacturer must be certain that his product meets the standards of identity if he labels in this way. Such federal regulations are intended to guide consumers at the grocery store.

There has been an interesting development related to labeling milk products and imitation milk products. Fresh whole milk must have a minimum of 3½ percent butterfat and 8.15 percent milk solids not fat. Fresh whole milk must meet the bacterial count standards required for Grade A milk. However, there are other imitation milk products available now that are competing for the usual milk market. These so-called filled milks may vary considerably from fresh whole milk, or they may simply be made by removing the butterfat and replacing this fat content with a vegetable fat.

The only way to get an idea as to what you are buying when you select a filled milk product rather than fresh whole milk is to *carefully read the label.* This will tell you the list of ingredients in the order of their weight in the product. You would certainly be wise to buy a product that lists nonfat milk or nonfat milk solids as a major ingredient if you decide to buy imitation milk. You will also find that some of the imitation milks are made from Grade B rather than Grade A quality milk. With so many new products such as these entering the market, it is important to form the habit of reading labels before buying.

There are many such choices confronting each shopper in the supermarket these days. Many of us can remember the time when the major decision about preparing breakfast was whether to slice or juice the fresh oranges. Today's shopper has the option of selecting fresh oranges, frozen orange juice concentrate, or synthetic orange drink.

ASCORBIC ACID ALTERNATIVES

From a nutritional standpoint, orange juice or one of its alternatives is a practical way of supplying the body's need for vitamin C, or ascorbic acid, every day. This naturally raises the question of what form of this product is best to buy. What's best can be interpreted in at least two ways—what tastes the best and what is best for your health. Taste is an individual matter. Many people prefer the taste of fresh oranges, but dislike the fuss involved in obtaining the juice for a family's breakfast needs. The convenience of the frozen concentrate has probably been instrumental in persuading many people that they prefer the concentrate. The synthetic orange drinks, yet another alternative, are preferred by others, presumably on the basis of cost, since fresh orange flavor has yet to be successfully reproduced synthetically.

One may get as much or more vitamin C from synthetic orange drinks than is in fresh orange juice because it is added. Frozen orange concentrate is comparable to the fresh juice not only in vitamin C, but also in carbohydrate, potassium and folic acid. Other minerals and vitamins are contained in trace amounts of both the frozen and fresh product. However, these nutrients are present in such small amounts compared with their quantities in many other foods that oranges are viewed as relatively unimportant sources for the other nutrients.

You should distinguish between synthetic frozen concentrates and various orangeades and pops. The latter are not intended to simulate full-strength orange juice and have at the most a very small amount of vitamin C added. In such a case, there is little nutritional value to the product. However, the synthetic products that are designed to simulate orange juice are excellent sources of synthetic vitamin C. Since the chemist has learned how to make vitamin C cheaper than oranges or grapefruit can make it, you usually get more nutrition for less money by buying the synthetic product. And, remember, synthetic vitamin C is identical to natural vitamin C in its nutritional properties.

Just as we have developed synthetic products containing vitamin C, there has been much success in fortifying or enriching a wide variety of products commonly found in the grocery store.

SOY FLOUR

Enrichment and fortification are terms familiar and synonymous to most consumers these days. We are accustomed to hearing of vitamin and mineral-enriched bread and cereals and fortified milk.

Another type of nutritional improvement is expanding—protein fortification or enrichment. One example of a superior, low-cost protein is soy flour. Although this product is not yet readily available to the housewife, it is widely used by manufacturers and processors to improve the protein quantity and quality of many prepared foods.

Most vegetable and cereal proteins are deficient in one or more of the essential amino acids required by the body for the synthesis of tissues and cells. These proteins do not support growth unless other proteins are present to supply the amino acids that are in short supply in the cereal proteins. Cereal proteins are known to be deficient in certain amino acids, particularly lysine, and are thus termed "incomplete" proteins. By adding soy flour, a vegetable protein of high nutritive quality, these amino acids that are low in the cereal protein are increased in the mixture. The combination of the two proteins tends to be "complete" and is thus more available for repair or synthesis of body cells.

Soy flour today bears little resemblance to that of several years ago. Improved technology has resulted in a product that can be combined easily with many types of food with only minor changes in taste and texture.

There are three types of edible soy flour: full-fat, which contains all of the natural fat of the soybean; low-fat, which has the fat content reduced to about 6 percent; and defatted, containing no more than one percent fat. The defatted soy flour is the one principally used by the baking industry and is available in granules ranging from coarsely ground grits to a fine powder similar to wheat flour.

Soy flour must be subjected to just the proper amount of treatment for its specific use. For maximum nutrition, soy flour must either be precooked or added uncooked to products that require long baking or cooking times. The uncooked flour is used to increase the protein content of breads, rolls, sweet doughs, and in dry mixes for cakes, muffins, and pancakes. A toasted soy flour is used in crackers, beverages, cookies, and cereals where the cooking time of the product is less, but where the slightly darker color of the toasted flour would not be noticeable.

Another food that has been a staple part of the diet for some races for centuries is now beginning to appear quite commonly on the American bill of fare. Since there are several products to choose from in the markets, it may be helpful to you to learn the nutritive merits of each type.

BUYING RICE

When you start to read labels on packages of rice, you may be surprised to discover the choices range from long grain to short, brown to polished, parboiled to enriched, and quick cooking to minute. The choices are wide, but the decisions are quite simple. There are three factors to consider: cost, nutritive value, and cooking time. For example, quick cooking and minute rices are convenient because they require very little preparation time. The disadvantages are that they are more expensive than the regular rices and the nutritive value is low.

A long time ago it was discovered that the brown, unpolished rice, which is high in thiamin, riboflavin, and niacin can be subjected to a short steaming process, which drives these B vitamins from the bran layer into the inner portion or endosperm of the rice kernel. Thus, when the brown layers of bran are removed from the rice grains, the B vitamins are retained in the portion of the cereal grain that is eaten. This parboiled rice is preferred by many because the nutritive value compares favorably with that of brown rice, but it cooks in about half the time required to soften the bran layer on brown rice and it has a longer shelf life than brown rice.

If you compare parboiled with polished rice (bran layer and germ have been removed, but with no steaming prior to the polishing), you find that parboiled rice is high in nutritive value compared with polished rice, because the vitamins are removed along with the bran layer in the processing of polished rice. As you would logically guess, the steam treatment required to preserve the nutritive value of parboiled rice does cost money, with the result that the price of parboiled rice is considerably higher than the polished counterpart.

By looking at samples of polished and parboiled rice side-by-side, you can notice a very slight difference in the appearance of the two types of rice. Polished rice is a snowy white, and parboiled rice is a slightly creamy color. This creamy or faintly yellow color is the proof positive that there has been a transfer of riboflavin, one of the desired B vitamins, from the bran to the main portion of the rice grain before the rice was polished. This faint yellow color is not undesirable, because it is actually unnoticeable unless you put the parboiled rice alongside polished rice. When seen alone, parboiled rice looks beautifully white. The higher nutritive value of parboiled rice makes this an excellent choice in the market despite its somewhat higher cost.

In a few places in this country and in several foreign countries, it is possible to buy enriched polished rice, which is a good source of the B vitamins and iron. Enriched rice is made by mixing polished rice with some other polished rice that has been coated with a vitamin premix. This vitamin premix can contain thiamin, riboflavin, niacin, and iron to supply the nutrients that were removed by the polishing process. When enriched rice is boiled in water, the vitamin premix will be dissolved into the cooking water and distributed throughout the rice you are cooking. This, of course, makes enriched rice another highly nourishing rice product you may wish to buy if it is available in your community.

Since parboiled, enriched, and brown rices are all good sources of the water-soluble B vitamins, it is important to prepare them in just enough water so that there is only a trace of moistness in the bottom of the pan when the rice is done. This keeps the vitamins in the rice you eat instead of in the water you throw down the drain.

As you well know, rice is only one of the cereal products available in the grocery store. When you get to the bread counter, you are well aware of the large number of choices that confront you there, and your choice may have a distinct bearing on the nutritive value of the product you carry home to your family.

A GLIMPSE OF THE BREAD COUNTER

Whole wheat bread has long been known to be a good source of thiamin, riboflavin, and niacin, three of the B vitamins that help to keep our nervous system in good shape, and fiber. These B vitamins, along with some minerals, are found in the bran layer surrounding the grain of wheat. The bran, as you will remember, is a light brown color and has a coarse texture. Both of these features make whole wheat products less pleasing to those people who prefer the color and softness of white bread. However, just look what happens when the bran layer is removed. If you take away the bran, you also remove those important B vitamins and minerals, leaving primarily a mixture of starch and protein in white flour. Bread made from this refined flour will give you calories from the starch and also a small amount of protein, but the important B vitamins have been lost.

Does this mean that you should never eat bread made with refined, white flour? White bread lovers will be pleased to know that most refined wheat flour has thiamin, riboflavin, niacin, and the mineral, iron, added to it. This enrichment of refined wheat flour is a real boon to you if you prefer white bread. Now you can get the nutrients you need in the bread of your choice. Of course, whole wheat bread is already a good source of these nutrients because the bran remains in whole wheat flour. Consequently, you will not find whole wheat flour with vitamins added to it. It does not need to be enriched.

The next time you go to the market, read the labels on the different kinds of bread. If your family prefers white bread, check to be sure that the brand you buy is made from enriched flour. The label on the loaf will tell you if the flour has been enriched. If there is nothing on the label that indicates that enriched flour with thiamin, riboflavin, niacin, and iron have been added, you would be wise to select a different brand of bread that does contain these nutrients. Since the law requires that the label must state when these nutrients have been added to flour, you know that white bread that is not labeled as enriched will be a poor substitute nutritionally for whole wheat bread.

Enriched white bread is a satisfactory substitute for the whole grain product. Two ounces (approximately two slices) of thin-sliced sandwich bread made with enriched flour will furnish a little more than ⅛th of your daily need for thiamin, seven percent of your riboflavin, about 12 percent of your niacin, and 10 percent of your daily iron requirement. That may seem to be a surprising contribution from a food that so many people feel is good only for filling you up. Just remember to be sure to buy enriched bread if you are selecting white bread.

BREAKFAST CEREALS IN PERSPECTIVE

We have had our choice of cereals from corn, wheat, oats, barley, and rice for many years. At one time the American public was contented with relatively simple, sometimes slightly dramatic processing techniques such as rolling, steel-cutting, or "shooting from guns." These products were considered to be the essential food at breakfast that children needed to stick to their ribs. These cereals are still available, of course, but today these traditional cereals are literally in the midst of a cereal explosion. Although this change is slightly less publicized than the population explosion, any mother who has threaded her way through this section of the store, accompanied by young children who have certain cereal coupons they need to send in for some cherished give-away item, will readily attest to the magnitude of the cereal selection problem.

If you start looking beyond the cartoons and coupons on the package, you will discover that cereals are emerging as highly nourishing foods, despite the processing and refining that some of them undergo. Many cereals are refined, which means that the bran layer, along with its vitamins, has been removed. This sounds like an unfortunate loss to our diets, but most cereals are now enriched. Enriched cereals have several vitamins added to them, and they also have iron added. If cereals have been enriched with these substances, this information is carried on the label. Some cereals are formulated to have an increased amount of protein. These cereals are marketed as high protein cereals and will usually cost somewhat more than other cereals. With the relatively high amount of protein in American diets, it is not essential to buy these high protein cereals, but they are a perfectly suitable choice if you like and can afford them, and wish to increase the protein content of your diet. Any of the bran-containing cereals, particularly those referred to as all-bran, are excellent sources of fiber.

Sugar-coated cereals have been criticized by some people because of the relationship of sugar to the incidence of dental caries. However, almost everyone puts sugar on cereals that are not already sugar-coated. In fact, some people pour far more sugar on their cereal than they would get on a sugar-coated product. The sugar-coated cereals have the advantage of having the sugar pre-measured so there is no possible conflict over the amount of sugar being added to the cereal. This can actually decrease calories for strong-minded youngsters who like to watch the sugar flow from the spoon to the cereal.

It has been shown that there is less likelihood of dental caries if teeth are brushed, or at least the mouth is rinsed well, each time a meal or snack is eaten. If this is done, sugar-coated cereals are a perfectly good choice for anyone who likes them. However, the answer to dental caries is not the elimination of sugar from cereals, or from the diet, but the fluoridation of community water supplies.

The wise shopper will check to see that the cereal selected is high in nutrients and one enjoyed by the family. It is a good idea to compare prices, at least among the various sizes of the preferred kind of cereal.

If you are a people watcher, you can learn a fair amount about their food habits and nutritional status. We are all aware when we see a fat person that he is eating more than his body needs for the work it is doing. There is another rather obvious, but considerably less common nutrition problem that is seen occasionally in the United States.

THE VALUE OF IODIZED SALT

At the turn of the century in inland areas of the United States and in the Pacific Northwest, the nutritional deficiency condition known as endemic goiter was causing considerable concern. People with this problem have an enlarged thyroid gland that is noticeable as a swelling at the front of the throat. Today this condition can be seen on occasion, but it is far less frequent than it was 75 years ago.

In case you are wondering what caused the reduction in endemic goiter, the answer is in the iodization of common table salt. Tests on the value of iodide in the diet were first carried out in Ohio, a portion of the Midwest which was commonly referred to at that time as the "Goiter Belt." Potassium iodide was added to the salt of an experimental group of teenagers to see if this substance had any effect on the development of goiter among this group. Teenagers were used because this seemed to be the age group most seriously afflicted with developing goiters. Just a small amount of this mineral was found to be needed to prevent goiter in almost all children. On the basis of this and similar important human nutrition studies, salt producers were authorized to add 0.01% of potassium iodide to table salt. This very small quantity of potassium iodide provided enough iodide to protect people from enlargement of the thyroid gland.

When you go to the store next time, notice the salt display. You will see two types of salt for your selection. There will be plain salt, and there will be other packages clearly labeled iodized salt. To protect yourself and your family against goiter, take the iodized salt home. The small amount of iodide you get in the salt you normally use each day is your protection against goiter. This is an insurance bargain you simply cannot afford to pass up, for the two types of salt are sold at the same price. This simple food additive, potassium iodide, is responsible for improving the appearance of many people and for increasing their productivity. People with endemic goiter not only are less attractive, but they also are usually rather tired and lack energy.

In earlier days, European royalty in some of the inland countries frequently had goiter. In fact, this was almost considered a mark of distinction, but today it is definitely viewed as a mark of poor nutrition. You may get some iodide from fish you eat, particularly from seafood, but to be really sure you are eating enough iodide, always buy iodized salt.

Milk is a rather perishable, but very important item in the diet. Usually it is rather convenient to use the fluid milk available via door-to-door delivery from the milkman or purchased in the grocery store. However, there are many times when it may be desirable to buy other milk products for economy's sake, for convenience, or for specific, unique uses.

MILK PRODUCTS FOR CONVENIENCE AND ECONOMY

Canned and dried milk products are handy to have on hand at all times. Both canned and dried milks have a long shelf life and can be stored easily on the shelf in a relatively cool, dry place until they are opened and ready to be used.

Thanks to modern development, nonfat dry milk solids are available at a very low cost compared to the price of fluid whole or even fluid skim milk. Of course, the dried milk is a great deal lighter to carry home than is the fluid counterpart, which is an advantage when shopping for a large family. Through research, manufacturers have now developed a skim milk powder that is very easily reconstituted, without the frustrating lumps that used to signal this product to consumers. If you feel the flavor of this dried product is less desirable than fluid whole or skim milk, it is still possible to save some money and modify the flavor by mixing the reconstituted nonfat dried milk solids with some fluid milk. When the mixture is chilled in the refrigerator, few people can tell the difference, but your pocketbook can.

Canned milks have been used extensively for many more years than the dried milks, but there still is some confusion in the minds of many about the difference between evaporated and condensed milk. Actually these are two very different products. Both evaporated and condensed milk are fluid milks marketed in cans, they are both rather thick as they come from the can, and they are both rather yellow liquids. However, if you look closer at both types of canned milk, you notice that the sweetened condensed milk is definitely thicker and slightly more creamy in appearance than the evaporated milk. Both types of milk are produced from fresh whole milk by evaporating about half of the water from the fresh milk. To make evaporated milk, manufacturers concentrate the milk by removing 60 percent of the water. This product is carefully sealed in a can and heat-treated to sterilize it. Vitamin D is often added to evaporated milk to improve its nutritional quality so that it will be comparable to vitamin D-enriched whole milk when it is diluted to its normal strength.

In contrast to evaporated milk, sweetened condensed milk is made by evaporating just about half the water from the whole milk and then adding a large quantity of sugar to keep the concentrated milk from spoiling in the can. It is this added sugar that makes sweetened condensed milk so different in its use from the canned evaporated milk. The shelf life of sweetened condensed milk is quite long, but gradually a chemical browning reaction between the added sugar and the concentrated protein in the milk begins to take place. The canned product will slowly turn a brown, caramel color and develop a caramel flavor. This caramelized, sweetened condensed milk is perfectly safe to eat. In fact, one use of sweetened condensed milk is as a caramel pudding. You can cause this natural chemical change to take place quite rapidly by heating the unopened can in a pan of boiling water rather than waiting for nature to take its course on the shelf.

Another interesting use of sweetened condensed milk is with an acid such as lemon juice. When lemon juice is added, the milk will quickly thicken without even being heated. Many desserts can be made using sweetened condensed milk in its condensed (rather than diluted) form, but this type of milk is not a good replacement for fresh milk as a beverage because of the high sugar content.

Many people are introduced to evaporated milk at a very early age because this canned milk is widely used as a base for preparing baby formulas in the home. This milk, which has a slightly cooked flavor, can be diluted with an equal amount of water to make a nutritionally satisfactory substitute for fresh milk. The undiluted evaporated milk is sometimes used in meat loaf, casseroles, and soups. If undiluted evaporated milk is chilled until ice crystals begin to form in it, you can whip this concentrated milk and use it as a replacement for whipping cream in desserts.

Along this same line, it is interesting to note some of the differences between ice cream and ice milk. First of all, there is little difference in the calorie content of the two products; although ice milk has less fat, it does contain more protein and carbohydrate than ice cream. The summary of the nutritional comparison of the two follows:

Nutrient	½ pint ice cream	½ pint ice milk
Calories	295	285
Protein	6 gm.	9 gm.
Fat	18 gm.	10 gm.
Carbohydrate	30 gm.	42 gm.

Consumers are also relieved of anxieties when they learn of some of the protective regulations in force to insure that the fresh, canned, and frozen meats in the grocery stores are safe to eat.

MEAT: EVEN SAFER THAN MEETS THE EYE

Remarkable progress has been made in the marketing of meat since the days when Upton Sinclair was writing about conditions in the meat industry. Now all meat that enters interstate commerce must be inspected for wholesomeness by federal inspectors. If the animal prior to slaughter is healthy and if the conditions following slaughter are maintained according to specified standards, each wholesale cut of the carcass will be stamped with a round seal that says U.S. Inspected and Passed. Poultry also are inspected and passing the inspection is usually indicated on a label attached to a wing. This stamp is your assurance that the food was safe at the time it was being held at the processing plant.

Federal legislation has made all states establish state laws that insure at least minimum standards comparable to the federal regulations for meat inspection on products that will be marketed within a state. Although some states previously had this type of legislation, the move will be a means of insuring sanitation of meats for all consumers, even when the meat does not cross state lines.

It may seem surprising when one considers how much meat is produced in this country, but imported meat products are currently enjoying a wide market here. To name a few, there are bacon from Canada, corned beef from Argentina, meatballs from Holland, dried sausage from Italy, and canned hams from Denmark. Each year we import meats from approximately 30 countries, and it is the job of the federal meat inspectors in the U.S. Department of Agriculture's Consumer and Marketing Service to be sure that these many products are all wholesome and safe to eat. Before either the frozen or processed meats can enter this country, they are carefully inspected. In fact, meat cannot even be shipped to the United States from another country until that country's meat inspection system has been found by our Department of Agriculture representatives to be comparable to our own inspection system.

The United States Department of Agriculture veterinarians regularly check these foreign inspection systems and their exporting plants to be sure that the products from other countries constantly meet the same standards of wholesomeness required of meat in this country. These foreign shipments of meat leave their original countries bearing an identification tag that gives pertinent information including a certification of inspection in the original country. When the meat arrives at a U.S. port, our own inspectors recheck each shipment. It is the inspector's responsibility to make five checks before a shipment is admitted. First, he must check the label against the one that has been officially approved. Then he checks the gross weight. Selected cans are emptied, washed and weighed to determine the net weight of the contents of the can. Of course, the meat product itself is carefully checked throughout to be certain that the product's characteristics agree with the description on the label. The actual wholesomeness of the meat is checked by sending randomly selected samples to the laboratory for careful chemical analysis.

Any meat shipments that do not pass this rigorous inspection are not admitted to the United States. Almost 3½ million pounds of canned meat were refused entry to this country in just one year.

Anytime you buy any imported meat or meat product, you will find it is prominently labeled as a product of the country from which it came. For instance, canned hams from Denmark will be conspicuously tagged as a product of Denmark. This is done as a matter of law, not necessarily as a matter of prestige. Thanks to the thorough inspection required for all imported meats, you can eat meats from any foreign country with the assurance that they are as safe to eat as the meat produced in the United States.

THE IMITATION CASE

"Things are not always what they seem," warned Gilbert and Sullivan in their operetta, "The H.M.S. Pinafore," and that saying certainly is appropriate in the food industry today. One product that may be creating considerable question in your shopping is the selection of modified and non-dairy products. Food technologists are unveiling all sorts of look-alikes, taste-alikes, smell-alikes, and so on.

Probably the most easily recognized is margarine. It is margarine which fought the battles of acceptance for many of today's substitute items. There are many of us who remember when margarine was sold as a white, lardy-looking substitute for butter, a far cry from the sophisticated products of today.

The dairy case today might almost be renamed the "imitation case" for it is full of many substitute or imitation products. Some of them are: creams, coffee whiteners, whipped toppings, modified sour creams, and non-dairy sour creams. They emerge in various forms—liquid, powdered, frozen, chilled, and spray (aerosol). The food chemists have been having a field day!

How are all of these dietary wonders performed? It makes one feel that eating has been transplanted from the dining room and kitchen to the chemistry laboratory. The basic ingredients in the imitation dairy products are fats, proteins, emulsifiers, stabilizers, flavors, colors, and water. Surely it is enough to give even the most modest cow an inferiority complex.

It is interesting to note that stabilizers and emulsifiers hold fat in suspension, stabilized as separate globules so the mouth feel is not oily. They also form emulsions with protein, preventing oil separation in whiteners for hot beverages and holding air in whipped or aerosol dispensed products. The label on a product may call a stabilizer and emulsifier exactly that, or may give the chemical names such as carrageenan, alginate, locust bean gum, etc.

Federal and state laws insure labeling with the components listed in order of quantity used, but the specificity may vary. One manufacturer may state simply vegetable oil, whereas another food processor will call it corn oil. Clearly, the specific identification of components provides the consumer with important information.

In some instances, the imitation product may be less expensive, have fewer calories, less fat or cholesterol, longer storage life, and may not require refrigeration. However, the consumer needs to weigh the advantages and disadvantages to himself carefully before blindly forsaking a quality product for an imitation simply because it is new.

These are only a few of the decisions faced by consumers when they are marketing for their groceries. To cover the subject completely would require a book just on that alone, but we hope we have given you a few useful tips in this chapter.

ALUMINUM: MENACE OR MAGNIFICENCE

The Food and Drug Administration reminds us that many old wives' tales still exist about the effect that cooking in various metal containers may have on health. The commonly used materials for cooking utensils include aluminum, alloys, glass, steel, tin, and cast iron, all of which are perfectly safe for general use. Although the cooking qualities of the various materials may have more appeal to one cook than to another, there appears to be no reason for refusing a pan made from the preferred material on the basis of health.

Aluminum is most frequently mentioned by consumers when they inquire about safety of pans. Every now and then consumers report efforts by salesmen of other types of cookware to try to convince them that cooking with aluminum is injurious to health.

The fact that aluminum utensils gradually become covered with a grayish substance which dissolves in boiling soda water or which can be rubbed off with a damp rag containing a pinch of soda is something demonstrated in their sales pitches as a way of suggesting that it would be consumed if soda is used in aluminum cookware. Actually, there is extensive evidence that cooking in aluminum utensils is harmless. The grayish coating which forms on these utensils is a harmless oxide or residue that is soluble in baking soda.

Aluminum occurs naturally in many foods. Also, aluminum compounds have a number of uses as direct food ingredients, for example in baking powders and in pickles to keep them firm. These uses are recognized as safe by scientists qualified to evaluate the safety of food additives.

Another common question is about frying pans coated with tough, white non-porous resins which permit the pan to be used for frying without adding shortening. These are advertised as a clean and desirable way to prepare diets low in fat. Data were submitted to the FDA to show the safety of such resins.

Some transfer of the utensil material to food occurs even with such a durable item as stainless steel. This quality is desirable in the case of cast iron skillets because the small amount of iron that transfers to food may be of value in supplying iron to the individual.

NUTRITION QUIZ

1. What is the cheapest source of the milk for your meals:
   a. Evaporated, b. Bottled, c. Dry
   Answer: Dry is correct. One of the best ways to cut costs without reducing food value is to use nonfat dry milk.
2. When oranges and orange juice are costly, which of the following is a good alternate source of vitamin C:
   a. ¾ cup canned grapefruit juice, b. 1½ cups tomato juice, c. 1⅓ cups shredded cabbage
   Answer: All three of these items are equal to one orange in vitamin C content. For an inexpensive source of this vitamin, just select the week's best bargain.
3. If you want an inexpensive source of iron, choose:
   a. Pork liver, b. Egg, c. Calf liver, d. Lamb liver
   Answer: You can buy whichever happens to be on special at the moment because all kinds of liver are abundantly supplied with iron, as well as a great number of other health builders. One egg makes a helpful contribution to an adult's daily iron requirement, but you can obtain 10 to 15 times more iron in three ounces of cooked liver.
4. Which is more economical: a. Large size packages and cans, b. Small containers
   Answer: Usually you will find that it is cheaper to purchase foods packed in large containers. However, do not be fooled by the appearance of the container, and do be sure that the one which looks larger actually holds more. Remember, too, that you are not being economical if some of the food spoils before it is used up. Be sure that if you buy a lot, you can either eat it all up or store it properly until it is all gone.
5. How would you rate these foods as good buys for vitamin A:
   a. Carrots, b. Greens, c. Sweet potato
   Answer: You will score high in this question if you know that you can choose the cheapest, because dark green and yellow vegetables are all

excellent sources of carotene from which we can make vitamin A. An adult's whole daily requirement of this important vitamin can amply be filled by ⅓-cup cooked carrots or spinach or other greens, or by one raw carrot or half a sweet potato. Squash is not quite so rich in carotene, but when it is inexpensive, it is a good buy, too.

6. Do you use the outer leaves of lettuce, cabbage, and broccoli?

Answer: We are pleased if you answered this one with a "yes." The dark green outer leaves of lettuce and cabbage and the leaves of broccoli are very high in vitamin A and more nutritious than the paler portions.

7

FUTURE, PAST, AND PRESENT TENSE

"No one will live all his life in the world to which he was born—and no one will die in the world in which he worked in his maturity." This statement was made some time ago by the late Dr. Margaret Mead, the well-known anthropologist. Dr. Mead continued,

> For those who work on the growing edge of science, technology, or the arts, contemporary life changes at even shorter periods. Often only a few months may elapse before something which was previously taken for granted must be unlearned or transformed to fit the new state of knowledge or practice. In today's world, no one can complete an education.

These comments certainly apply to food and nutrition, not only today, but in the recent and far distant past. Even in the days of primitive man, changes took place, especially after the discovery of fire when man learned to cook his food. Somewhere along the way man learned to preserve food by drying, smoking, and salting.

Many generations after the discovery of fire, man developed practical agriculture. This progressed very slowly, but brought about enormous changes which have been going on ever since. Agriculture enabled man to forsake a nomadic life, and as vast areas of hunting lands were eliminated and the huntsman found fewer and fewer animals, the importance of the new foods produced by agriculture became more apparent and accepted. Naturally, there were tremendous changes in food habits.

Getting to more recent times, there have been tremendous technological changes in agriculture since the middle 1800's. Much of this stems from President Lincoln's interest in agriculture and the establishment of our land grant

157

colleges, for in these institutions agricultural research, technology, and education have developed and flourished.

Before the scientific revolution in agriculture and food sciences, we were troubled because our food needs were not always met. Today, in our country, we are troubled with the perplexities of exceeding the food requirements for feeding our own nation, improving nutrition practice, and sharing food surpluses and technologic know-how with others.

There is always the reality of nutritional improvement of basic and indigenous foods with synthetic nutrients. The addition of iodine to salt and vitamin D to milk are classic examples of foods indigenous to the U.S. diet. The addition of the synthetic amino acid, lysine, to wheat products to turn an inadequate protein into one that is nutritionally adequate is important in improving nutrition in several countries of the world today.

Actually, totally synthetic foods are possible and may someday be vital in feeding the world. All known nutrients can be made synthetically. The important challenge is how to put these nutrients together to make a synthetic food that is palatable for those who are to eat it. As Dr. Emil Mrak, former Chancellor of the University of California at Davis, pointed out, synthetic foods will have to taste, smell, broil, and thrill equally as well as those produced by nature if they are to be successful.

The introduction of new food has had, and will continue to have, historic and political significance. The introduction of the potato and corn into Europe are classic examples.

OF CORN AND POTATOES

Today the potato not only contributes nutritionally to the diets of many countries, but has led a most fascinating march through the economic and social history of many lands.

The Spanish conquerors of Peru brought the potato back to Europe when they returned in the 15th century. As with much that is new, potatoes were regarded for some time with suspicion in many places. However, when they were introduced to the Irish, reportedly by Sir Walter Raleigh, the Irish took to this food with alacrity because of necessity. They nourished themselves and they fattened their pigs on this New World food. The potato became so deeply entrenched in the eating pattern of the Irish peasant population that other basic foods were neglected. For example, corn and corn meal were offered to much of the starving population during the Irish famine of the mid-19th century, but there was no means of milling the corn, and women had no knowledge of cooking corn products, so corn actually did little to alter the course of the famine.

The acceptance of the potato by the English took time, and it was many years before the potato became daily fare in England. Frederick the Great introduced the potato to the Germans during a famine in 1774, but it was promptly rejected. Later he overcame this opposition by teaching the people how to cultivate and use potatoes. Potatoes were grown on his own private lands and consumed by the royal family.

Corn also has an important social and nutritional history. It is generally accepted that corn is a new world product and that it was introduced into Europe at the end of the 15th century. Corn is often referred to as "Indian corn" in Europe, particularly in England. In many instances, corn has been considered a poor man's cereal and as such was not well received as a human food by northern Europeans. It did, however, become a staple in Spain, Portugal, Rumania, and Hungary.

New foods or augmenting the supply of familiar foods is still making history and influencing social and economic development. Shipping millions of tons of nonfat dry milk to developing countries has tremendous implications for history in the making, as does the rapidly expanding soybean industry. The controversy over the manufacture of fish meal for human consumption has political, as well as nutritional significance.

Whether you think of the tomato as the romantically titled "love apple" or simply as something really good to eat, we think you will find this brief quiz on tomatoes interesting.

ANYONE FOR LOVE APPLES?

1. How one classifies tomatoes is a frequent cause of disagreement. In fact, the law had to come into the matter at one time. What is your opinion?

   a. Fruit; b. Vegetable

   Answer: If you checked either fruit or vegetable, you would be correct. Botanically, the tomato is a fruit, but by legal action it is a vegetable. In 1893, the United States Supreme Court decided that, because it was served with the main part of the meal, the tomato was a vegetable. This was all because of an import duty suit.

2. What vitamins are tomatoes particularly noted for contributing to our daily needs?

   a. Vitamin A, b. Riboflavin, c. Vitamin C, d. Vitamin D

   Answer: a and c. Tomatoes are an excellent source of the provitamin A substance called carotene. One small tomato will have about 1100 International Units of vitamin A as carotene—about ⅕ of the recommended daily intake. Tomatoes are also a good source of vitamin C—approximately 25 milligrams per tomato. This amount represents almost half of the recommended allowance. Tomatoes are not a good source of riboflavin and contain little, if any, vitamin D.

3. Which of the following products is the most nutritious?

   a. Raw tomatoes, b. Canned tomatoes, c. Tomato juice

   Answer: All three styles of tomatoes are very similar in most of the important nutrients. Both canned tomatoes and tomato juice are usually found to have lost some vitamin C in the canning process, but these products are still very good sources of this vitamin as well as vitamin A (carotene).

4. What is the origin of the tomato?

Spain, France, The Garden of Eden, Peru, England, Italy

Answer: Supposedly, the tomato originated in Peru, was introduced in Europe by the Conquistadores, and became popular in the United States because of an interest in things French. In Mrs. Emma Weigley's story of tomatoes (*Journal of the American Dietetic Association,* February, 1964), it was reported that colonial Americans probably knew about the tomato, but considered it to be poisonous or an aphrodisiac. In the 1818 edition of the *American Gardener* is found the earliest surviving recipe for tomato catsup.

Thoughts of catsup quickly turn one's mind to food in the army or other military service.

A HISTORICAL GLIMPSE OF FOOD TO CONQUER THE WORLD

"An army travels on its stomach" is a well known axiom. In another sense, this applies to civilians, too, because advances in the feeding of soldiers almost always lead to new and useful convenience foods for everyone. All of us directly or indirectly benefit from improvements in the foods of the armed forces. Research that makes this possible is done by the Quartermaster Research and Engineering Command working with a special advisory council of the National Academy of Sciences. Some of their developments make interesting reading.

Food for the military is certainly not a new idea. Five thousand years ago the Egyptians realized that their troops could not go far unless equipped with food that was able to travel. They invented bread, and ever since, it has been termed "the staff of life" both in and out of the army.

Another product we take for granted also was born of the necessities of war. When Napoleon sent out an SOS for a method of food preservation that would enable his navy to stay well fed at sea, one bright Frenchman came up with the can. Through most of history, however, military forces were not well fed. When the Athenians and Spartans were warring against each other in ancient Greece, time had to be called every noon so that ships could be beached and the sailors could go to town for lunch. Centuries later, U.S. soldiers in the Civil War had to supplement their scanty food supplies by foraging on the land.

Even as recently as World Wars I and II, army food was not exactly popular. Now different types of meals are being developed so that a soldier in every conceivable situation will have food that is quick and easy to prepare, boosts his efficiency and morale, and is as attractive and tempting as possible.

The first type, a ready-to-eat meal, is separately packaged for use by an individual soldier. In a light-weight, flexible container he will have food that will be tasty even when cold and that can be eaten under the most difficult conditions. Not hash, mind you, but chicken leg or sliced steak, shrimp with sauce, peaches or pineapple or blueberries!

For conditions in which some preparation is possible, there are heat-and-eat meals needing little equipment. Cleverly designed containers serve both as cooking utensils and dishes. Hot water and 20 minutes are the only requirements for preparing this meal. Gone are the poor powdered eggs and potatoes of the past. Modern methods of vacuum drying and freeze-drying have replaced such early products with steaks and chops and even French-fried foods.

Much has changed even in the ready-to-cook meals for rear areas where cooking facilities and personnel are available. Radiation preservation, instead of heat, to prevent food spoilage, has been used to make available a large selection of prefabricated, uncooked meals, and a fabulous variety of near-fresh foods such as turkey and ham. There is even a remarkable bread mix that actually permits fresh baked bread in rear combat zones.

New techniques by the Quartermaster Corps have contributed to the bright nutritional future for all of us. It is to another nation's navy that we owe early recognition of the value of citrus fruits in preventing scurvy.

MEET THE LIMEYS

If you have been laboring under the illusion that the British sailors got the name of "limey" because they turned green when the ships started to roll, this true story is especially for you.

Actually, we owe a debt to the British sailors and others who used to go on very long ocean voyages. Before this century, refrigeration and effective means of storing food for long periods of time were practically unknown. Consequently, people sailing across the oceans for weeks and even months had a very limited diet of staples and little else. This was unfortunate, but it did help a few keen observers to develop the idea that health is related to the food you eat. These early adventurers usually suffered from impaired health as well as the rigors of the trip itself. Early sailors developed painfully swollen gums that bled easily; their teeth often loosened and some fell out. A few people even died as their symptoms became worse. Finally in the mid-1800's, the British naval officers decided that they would have to try to improve the health of their sailors, and they hit upon the idea of trying to do this by changing the food available on the ships. Of course, they still carried a large supply of staple foods, but in addition, the ships were stocked with a good supply of limes and other citrus fruits. Interestingly enough, this addition of fresh citrus fruit to the ship's fare remarkably improved the health of the sailors. Their gums remained healthy and showed no tendency to become inflamed and swollen. As a result of this experiment, all the ships in the British navy were required to carry limes and other citrus fruits. This practice, of course, quickly resulted in people tagging British sailors with their nickname of "limey," and the name has stuck down through the years.

At the time it was discovered that citrus fruits had this mysterious power to prevent scurvy, nutrition was not the science it is today. No one knew what there was about citrus fruits that protected the sailors. They simply observed that eating these fruits made a difference in the health of the men. Now we know that the mysterious substance is vitamin C or ascorbic acid. The mystery is gone. The only mystery that remains today is why some people still develop early symptoms of scurvy when we have knowledge of the vitamin and its numerous food sources. In all locales in the United States, there are abundant supplies of foods that provide this important vitamin, but there are still a few people who either are not aware of the need for this vitamin, who cannot afford, or who do not select diets containing foods rich in vitamin C.

You can be sure you are eating this important vitamin if you include a citrus fruit in your diet each day. Citrus fruits are good sources of ascorbic acid, and they are readily available all year long. Of course, habits today are different from those of a few years back, and our habits with citrus fruits have changed some, too. Fortunately, frozen orange juice is an excellent source of vitamin C, so you don't have to prepare fresh oranges unless you want to. For variety, try strawberries, tropical fruits, or plenty of cabbage or potatoes, and don't forget tomatoes. All of these add to your vitamin C intake.

An American researcher named Crandon did some important research on vitamin C in this century to help illustrate why this vitamin was important to good health.

CRANDON AND COLLAGEN

Some people swallow vitamin C tablets by the handful when they have a cold in the vain hope that it will miraculously cure them. Others are aware that ascorbic acid is a vitamin, but have never worried greatly about what this particular vitamin does for them. However, largely through the work of Crandon, we know that vitamin C is necessary for the formation of collagen, the connective tissue needed for healing cuts and scratches. Crandon, using himself as the experimental subject, demonstrated his theory that vitamin C plays a role in wound healing. He first ate a diet that was very low in ascorbic acid to make his body be depleted of this vitamin. Then some cuts were made in his back. In a well-nourished person, we would expect collagen to form rather quickly and close the wound. However, the cuts on Crandon's back simply did not heal. They remained as open as they were the day he made them. No new connective tissue was forming to knit the wound back together. After several days, it was apparent that his wound was not improving, so he then began to eat foods that were good sources of vitamin C. Sure enough, the cuts began to heal as the level of this vitamin built up in his body once again.

Certainly this scientist showed a remarkable degree of devotion to his science to prove his theory about the wound-healing function of ascorbic acid.

One common reason for low vitamin C intake in the United States is the problem of breakfast skipping. Orange juice and other citrus products are mostly likely to be served on the breakfast menu. If this meal is skipped, it is reasonable to expect that the intake of vitamin C will be low. Another reason for inadequate vitamin C is its instability or rapid loss from foods. When vitamin C is exposed to air, it is quickly changed to a related compound that does not possess the activity of the vitamin. To protect the vitamin C content of foods rich in this substance, avoid exposing these foods to air until just before serving. Oranges are best sliced just before they are served, and so are grapefruit. By keeping cut surfaces to a minimum, you also help to retain more of this elusive vitamin. For example, whole fresh strawberries are higher in vitamin C than are sliced fresh berries.

Your daily need for vitamin C can be provided by drinking six ounces of orange juice. Or maybe you would like a more exotic source such as half a papaya to provide your daily vitamin C quota. Two medium tomatoes, ⅔ of a cup of turnips, ½ cup of broccoli, or ⅔ cup of Brussels sprouts are also ways of getting the vitamin C you need.

Now let's glance briefly at a nutrition problem that was urgent in the United States at the turn of the century.

PELLAGRA IN PERSPECTIVE

It has always been possible to find isolated cases of malnutrition in the United States as well as in any other country of the world because there are always people who are not eating a good diet. The reasons for their malnutrition may be quite varied. It may be that there is simply not enough understanding of what to eat to be well-nourished. Some people are malnourished because they have learned to like only a few foods. In other cases economic crises within the family or the country may make it impossible for a family to be well fed. All of these factors help to explain the malnourished around the world.

In our country there was a vitamin-deficiency condition that was an all-too-common problem in the South during the 19th and early 20th centuries. This condition was called pellagra, and it was a particular problem among that populaton that ate a great deal of corn and had little meat in the diet. These people developed symptoms that are sometimes referred to as the "three D's"—diarrhea, dermatitis, and dementia. One of the unique things about this condition was that the dermatitis affected comparable areas on both sides of the body. This was called "symmetrical dermatitis." For instance, it was common for a rash to develop on both hands or on both elbows, as well as other spots on the body. As the disease progressed, the mind was often affected and did not function normally. If the condition was not treated, it was likely to become more serious, and many people did die from pellagra. We now know that this condition is caused entirely by a dietary deficiency. The missing nutrient in pellagrous patients is niacin, one of the B vitamins. If patients are treated with this vitamin, they usually will begin to recover from this dreadful condition.

Pellagra can be avoided in the first place simply by eating an adequate diet that is rich in niacin (as well as other nutrients needed for good health). Our best practical sources of niacin are all types of meats. Beef is high in niacin. Pork is also a suitable food to provide niacin. Lamb is even higher in this important B vitamin than are pork and beef. Don't overlook fish as an important source of niacin in your diet. Milk is not very high in niacin, but it is an excellent potential source of this vitamin: milk contains an abundance of an amino acid called tryptophan, and your body can convert tryptophan from milk and other foods into the niacin it needs. Consequently, you can consider milk as an important food to help supply niacin. A few vegetables and fruits are fair sources of niacin or tryptophan, but many of them such as corn are very low in both of these substances.

For a change of pace, let's see how food habits and nutritional status have influenced our ideas of beauty through the ages.

CHANGING PORTRAITS

It is interesting to look back through history to see what art can reveal to us about nutritional status in ages past. For example, in classic Greek sculptures you will begin to see what we mean when we say that nutrition and beauty are related. If you have been constantly battling your weight to try to achieve the slim, sylph-like figure so popular today, you may look with an appreciative and sympathetic eye at the various Greek statues so commonly endowed with the well-rounded curves that can also be achieved today simply through too much food and too little exercise. Perhaps you are even comforting yourself with the thought that you really are just the right weight, the problem simply is that you were born in the wrong period of history. Think how favorably you would have been looked upon if you had had the foresight to arrive on earth during that era!

Fortunately, today's statistics tell us that you will be more likely to live longer if you avoid the extra curves caused by excess fatty deposits.

For another example of nutrition and art, look at paintings of the royal families of central Europe, such as those in Austria. Do you notice the scarf so commonly used to strategically cover the enlarged lump on the front of the throat? Some paintings even show this growth as a symbol of beauty and prestige. We know today that this enlargement on the front of the throat so common in medieval times was not a symbol of royal birth or special knowledge. It simply was a very noticeable sign that these people were not getting enough iodide in their diets, with the result that they developed a goiter, or an enlarged thyroid gland. This was found in central Europe because the diets in inland regions did not include fish from the sea that would have supplied the necessary iodide to prevent goiter.

For an example closer to home, let's look at paintings of women in the colonial days of America. The one condition common to almost all of the paintings from this period in history is the paleness of the skin. Poets ecstatically described the fairness of the skin as though this were a mark of distinction to be highly prized. Indeed, very pale skin was considered to be highly desirable at that time. It is apparent to nutritionists, however, that the women of colonial times were probably anemic as a result of eating too little meat to supply the iron they needed to maintain the desirable hemoglobin level in their blood. The outward visible sign was the very pale skin of these delicate ladies. Stories of this era bear out this conclusion. Women seemed to need to be treated with considerable care lest they faint, and ladies of wealth certainly were not expected to carry out physical labor of any type. We know today that when dietary intake of iron is low, the skin will appear to be pale and the body will be tired.

Thus, you can see through the Greek statuary, paintings of medieval royalty in Europe, and paintings and literature of colonial times that diets have been lacking in different nutrients. Eating for good health requires a combination of today's science and an appreciation of the artistic aspect of foods.

THE BRILLIANT BRILLAT-SAVARIN

You and your health are affected in many ways by your nutrition. To be well and strong, you have to have the right amounts of the right foods. Yet you need something more, too. True, food nourishes the body in a physical way, but it also nurtures the spirit. For best results, the rules for good nutrition have to be seasoned by recipes for good eating.

The experts at this important combination are the gourmets. For them, eating is a ceremony, food an artistic creation, and meals long and leisurely. Famous among these gourmets was the Frenchman, Jean-Anthelme Brillat-Savarin. He was a remarkable gentleman, and his fascinating life was as rich and varied as the meals he relished.

Brillat-Savarin was born in France in 1755 into a well-to-do family. He became a lawyer, but he found time for many other interests. He delved into medicine and music, chemistry and hunting, and above all into the secrets of the kitchen. He dined in the best homes and inns of the land and learned the finest wines, the most subtle seasonings, the rarest foods and recipes. All this came to an abrupt end when the French Revolution forced Brillat-Savarin to flee his native land. Then his many interests and talents became his salvation. They enabled him to overcome obstacles which would have crushed a less resourceful person.

Seeking a haven in America, he set sail for Boston. There he astounded that Puritan town by introducing a new dish, a fondue, in the city's most fashionable

restaurant. This caused a sensation and earned him the chef's richest reward—
a fresh-killed deer. Later, in New York City, he supported himself by giving
French lessons and by playing first violin in the city's only theater orchestra.
For diversion he went hunting in Connecticut and once spent days preparing
a wild turkey for the enjoyment of his American guests.

After the Revolution, Brillat-Savarin returned to France to spend the last 25
years of his life developing his spectacular array of abilities. In addition to his
legal work, he wrote on many subjects and finally at 70 produced his famous
book *The Physiology of Taste*. In this witty commentary on the pursuit of
happiness, Brillat-Savarin meditated on people, on food, and on fine eating.
Some of his comments could have been taken from yesterday's newspaper.
An appropriate example is this quotation, "For to be exactly stout enough,
neither too much nor too little, is for women the study of their life."

Notes to the men, too, also sound modern and useful in our own overfed
United States. Brillat-Savarin warned that danger lies in wait for the men who
eat "as long as they feel hungry, in spite of doctors." Though dining was his
supreme pleasure, this famous gourmet realized the wisdom of restraint. He
even formulated three rules for "overcoming corpulence: discrimination in
eating, moderation in sleep and exercise on foot or horseback." Good rules
for the 1980s!

8

NUTRITION: PROBLEMS IN AND OUT OF THIS WORLD

Humanity is sorely pressed. We all know about missiles and bombs and nuclear war, but there is another danger equally serious although it occupies the headlines only occasionally. Well-informed and responsible professionals are alerting the world to the fact that—starvation may destroy the human race.

Incredible? Yes, it is to us in our wonderfully fertile United States. It is not incredible, though, to the billions who wake up hungry every single day. Two-thirds of the world's population are ill and weak because they never get enough to eat.

This is an old story—from stone age to steel age, man has always been haunted by fear of famine. Now the world's population is multiplying at an all-time high, so it has become an even more staggering job to feed the world's people.

Even far back in the ice age food was scarce. In those remote times, twenty square miles of hunting grounds were required to feed just one family group. And variety of fare was certainly not the spice of life. One single animal was a grocery store, butcher shop, and department store all rolled into one. The all-purpose reindeer was sole supplier of the material for food and shelter, clothing and weapons. Interestingly, today there are still Lapps who spend their lives following the reindeer across the top of the world. In other parts of the world, though, man tired of roaming and started the shift from food gathering to food producing. As long as 6,000 years ago, in Egypt and the Middle East groups of people began to settle down and raise cattle, sheep, swine, water buffalo, and fowl. Life was a precarious day-to-day existence. In times of plenty, everyone gorged; in times of scarcity, they starved. Only after countless famines did it occur to someone to try to store for tomorrow what he could not eat today.

Gradually over centuries there developed ways and means of preserving and storing surpluses. At first, food was dried in the hot sun and wind; soon it was also preserved by smoking and salting. All through the Middle Ages poor folks survived by using salted foods. Then, less than 200 years ago, Englishmen thought of using ice to preserve fish. About the same time, a Frenchman first discovered a way to save surpluses by preserving and canning.

Though refrigeration and frozen foods are common household items in this country now, machinery for artificial refrigeration was not invented until about 1850. Finally, the most recent step in this long, slow development has been the use of chemicals for preserving food. Enormous advances have been made just in the 20th century.

Yet the task is far from complete. Tools and teaching, new chemicals, great imagination, and dedicated workers are needed. The billions who are still hungry must learn up-to-date methods of production and preservation. The millions being born each year must be fed from still unused lands and unexplored seas, from better crops and new foods.

At the United Nations 2500 workers are spending some 50 million dollars a year in this gigantic battle, not much considering the magnitude of the problem. There is no time to waste. All of us must combine our efforts if our world is to conquer hunger before hunger conquers us!

The world could benefit greatly from the application of the expertise of some of the displaced logistics experts (the so-called "bean counters") of the aerospace industry to the solution of closing the gap between the mushrooming population and providing an adequate food supply.

STARVATION: PARTIALLY A LOGISTICS PROBLEM

Will the world be able to grow enough food to feed enough people fast enough, and will enough people learn fast enough to make the best use of the available food?

The magnitude of this question almost defies the imagination, because the dimensions have been set by the population explosion. From the birth of the first man back in pre-historic times until 1850 the world produced only one billion people. Now, only 100 years later, there are already three billion people, and by the year 2000 even this staggering number will be doubled! Less than thirty years from now six billion individuals will be competing for the earth's food. How can we make sure there will be enough and that it will be wisely used?

These enormous problems are subjects for much thought, both by experts in the field and by the lay public. Certainly the biggest challenge is providing food for the underfed four-fifths of the world, even though significant strides have been made. In addition, there are concerns regarding nutrition even in areas of the U.S. which might be described as regions with a food surplus. As the nation has discovered, there is plenty of poor nutrition in our country. The problem generally is not food shortages, but frequently the failure of people to eat enough of the right foods for good health. Insufficient income or poor use of food money, stubborn adherence to old habits, and fondness for food fads are keeping millions of people ill-fed and under par.

Nutritionists, educators, doctors, and dentists are uniting their efforts to improve nutrition in this country. However, the task is immense and unfortunately, there simply are not enough professionals trained in this area. In the end, "sub par" nutrition in the United States will only be eradicated when everyone, you and your family and all of our citizens, realize that health and national productivity can definitely be improved by eating the right food. How can we, as nutritionists, persuade you, the public, to give up old habits when they are detrimental and to adopt new habits if they promise better health? Perhaps some of you readers have suggestions? In universities, in federal and state agencies, and in business, men and women are striving to make good nutrition a reality for everyone. The rest is up to you!

A GLIMPSE OF PROGRESS ON THE FARM

A newscaster was heard to say that a study on starvation and its effects was being planned, but that the study could not be conducted here because no real pocket of starvation could be found in the United States.

That simple statement is one of the many unheralded triumphs of science. While half the world goes to bed hungry every night, there is no concentrated area of starvation in our country. True, we have thousands of Americans with inadequate diets, but starvation of large numbers of people has not occurred in America for many, many years.

There are two other factors to look at. One is that fewer farmers with less arable land feed more people every year. The second is that the food in our country costs a smaller percent of our income than anywhere else in the world.

Take the first factor. About sixty years ago we had 13½ million agricultural workers feeding over 95 million people. Today, fewer than six million farm workers feed 183 million people. Part of the reason is the increased mechanization of farms, with machinery doing in a fraction of the time what it took hand labor many hours to do. But the rest of the picture, so often missed, is that agricultural chemicals have increased the productivity of farms by nurturing the soil and by controlling pests. Without these chemicals, Americans would have neither the abundance nor the variety of food that we enjoy.

As to the cost of food, we spend about 21% of our income for food, compared with the Peruvian housewife who spends 40%, the Japanese spending 42%, the West German's 45%, or the Soviet Union's 56% of the paycheck, and these figures are before the recent rise in food prices!

What you can't see on any chart or graph is the quality of the food we eat. Wormy applies were commonplace when many of us were children. You scarcely ever see a wormy apple any more. White bread is more nutritious than ever before in history, thanks to the chemicals (nutrients) that are added through enrichment to fortify the bread. Chemicals have taken up where nature left off to help make us among the healthiest people in the world.

With our population increasing daily and with millions of people looking to us for bare subsistence, or in some instances seeking our knowledge of scientific farming methods, science has new frontiers to conquer in the next few decades. We will need more food from less land and fewer farmers. And we will continue to demand better food at prices we can afford. The miracle is that we will probably get it.

Our nation has long been concerned with the problem of feeding its people well. Legislation at the national level has contained provisions through the years to aid in meeting this goal. Indicators of this concern are the legislation concerning the school lunch programs and the program of food stamps.

A SMATTERING OF HISTORY

This country has a heritage of seeking ways for improving the lot of man, and since its founding, improvement in agriculture and food supply has always been a major concern. About 120 years ago, during the time of the Civil War, Congress passed the Morrill Act. This Act gave emphasis to the agricultural and the mechanical arts, and from this developed our great colleges and universities that are called "land grant institutions." Also, the Agricultural Extension Service was given the charge to bring scientific information into the farm and the home. President Lincoln recognized the importance of agriculture and nutrition in all its ramifications for progress in the United States.

Since Lincoln's day the discipline of nutrition has been found to have increasingly broad and vital influence on the health patterns of entire nations, on the processing of foods, on the growing of crops, on the laws of government and international agencies, and lastly on our personal health. The nutritional status of the people of the world is intrinsically related to local food habits, traditions, the state of agriculture, and political and social conditions.

At a time when half the world's children are in need of calories and protein foods and a time when the other half faces overnutrition which favors the development of many of our common causes of ill health—at a time when half the world's adults are in need of more to eat to provide energy for increased productivity and hope for a better world, and the other half face diseases related to arteriosclerosis of largely unknown origin, except as connected to overeating and poorly balanced nutrition—food becomes increasingly important in our civilization. Just a few weeks before his assassination, President Kennedy addressed the Centennial Convocation of the National Academy of Science. He was just as concerned with agriculture and food production as was

President Lincoln a hundred years before; however, he emphasized food production and utilization as a *world problem*. In his speech, President Kennedy said:

> The earth can be an abundant mother to all of the people that will be born in the coming years if we learn to use her with skill and wisdom, to heal her wounds, replenish her vitality and utilize her potentials. . . . This seems to me the greatest challenge to science in our time to use the world's resources to expand life and hope for the world's inhabitants.

We have the responsibility to help move our society and the society of the entire world to a new era—an era which will reduce hunger and increase health and well being. We cannot do this alone; international cooperation is essential. Again quoting President Kennedy, "I particularly solicit your help in meeting a problem of universal concern—the supply of food to the modern world."

Let us implant ideas of good nutrition that will take root. Let us use our knowledge and apply nutrition so that our knowledge and skills will help create a world of peace, health, and well-being.

Largely as a result of governmental concern about feeding our citizens well, there has been systematic collection of data summarizing the consumption patterns of Americans over an extended period of time. From these data, we learn some interesting and useful facts about our food habits.

FOOD CONSUMPTION: USA

We are always being told that habits, particularly food habits, are hard to change. No doubt this is true, especially in terms of days and even weeks. Any reducer can attest to the problems of confronting a whole new pattern for eating. And we have all heard the wails of the housewife who can't get her "meat and potatoes" eating husband to branch out a bit and try some vegetables and salads.

However, over the years the American diet has changed and changed a lot. The U.S. Department of Agriculture has compiled some interesting figures. For example, we use half as much wheat and wheat products and potatoes now as we did in 1889, a decline from about 220 pounds per person annually to about 110 pounds. In the same period our consumption of sugars and syups has more than doubled—from 52 pounds per person in 1889 to 120 pounds in 1981. And 60 or 70 years ago we ate 16 times as much corn products as we do now. So while we diet-conscious ones have cut down on cereals and potatoes, we have developed (or indulged) our sweet tooth.

We eat more fruits and vegetables (except for potatoes) than we did at the turn of the century. While overall fruit consumption has gone up by 10 to 15 percent in the past 50 years, there has also been a big shift from apples to oranges and a shift from fresh to processed fruit. In 1889 we crunched our way through 107 pounds of apples a year, almost an apple a day. In the 1970s the amount was only 26 pounds. In the same period, we changed from 18 pounds to 79 pounds of citrus fruits.

And what about meat? While we don't eat quite as much protein as we did in 1900, a lot more of it comes from meat and less from cereals. We eat more eggs, more milk, more beef, and about twice as much poultry now. The chicken figures are almost spectacular! Sixty years ago Americans ate about 16 pounds of poultry per person a year. By 1961 the figures were 38 pounds and are continuing to rise.

We now get more of our calories from fat (about 41 percent) than we did in the first decade of this century. Then, fat contributed only about 32 percent of the total calories. But there is something rather interesting about this fat story. While our overall fat intake has increased, the increase has been through the use of margarine and other vegetable oils. There has been little or no increase in animal fat—just a shift in sources to provide a little less fat from butter to a little more from meat.

So we have made some really major changes in the way we eat, and this was done without really thinking about it. While it is useful to know that food habits can be changed, it is also wise to see whether the change has been for the better. A quick tour of the world, beginning with the United States, will give you a bit more insight into the nutrition problems of the 80's.

AMERICANS, THE BEAUTIFUL?

For years we have thought of America as the land of wealth and plenty, where crops always grow well, and all the people can have all the food they want to eat. In such a country, surely all the inhabitants are well fed, or are they?

The word "malnourished" is used to describe people who are not fed as well as they could be. Usually, when you hear the word malnutrition, you envision a group of starving children with sad faces and sharply protruding bones. Have you ever stopped to think that in many parts of the United States we do indeed have nutrition problems? You are constantly surrounded by malnourished people in the United States, but many of them are people suffering from over-nutrition rather than under-nutrition. In other words, they are plump or fat because they have been eating more food than their bodies need. This is the number one nutrition problem in the United States today! Over-nutrition is caused by a combination of changes in our society. Today we have discretionary income after the necessities of life are provided, and many people choose to spend this "extra" money for more food than they actually need for good nutrition. Another reason so many Americans are over-nourished is that we have so many machines to do our work that we are not nearly as active physically as people were at the turn of the century. As a result, we really should not eat so much food to keep our bodies going. Unfortunately, tempting foods are becoming increasingly easier to prepare and more available as the range of convenience foods is expanded. Now, if you couple this ready-to-eat food supply with the inertia and boredom stemming from an evening of sedentary television entertainment, you find that the most interesting and absorbing thing to do is to sit and eat. The ready availability of food, the decrease in physical activity, and today's prosperity are combining to turn us into an over-weight, over-nourished society.

A second problem we have is the large amount of saturated fat we eat. This excess fat tends to make us too heavy and also increases the likelihood of developing heart disease. You are probably thinking that you really don't eat very much fat, but let's just check and see where you might find fat that you were not aware of. Deep-fat fried foods of all types are popular in our culture. French-fried potatoes and potato chips are two of the most popular snack foods, and they are both excellent sources of fat. Salad dressings can do amazing things to the fat intake of the dieter. Meats are the major source of fat. Remember, it isn't just the butter or margarine you spread on your bread that puts fat in your diet. The hidden sources of fat are important.

Many people in America were shocked to learn in 1969 that hunger existed in America. It was a horrible revelation to see babies who had been fed so poorly that they weighed less when they were one year old than they did when they were born. In some families, people are poorly fed because they simply cannot buy enough food for everyone to eat well. Public pressure has helped to make surplus commodities and food stamps available to these families to at least partially supply their nutritional needs. However, the best nutrition can be obtained for our entire country only when all people have the opportunity to learn what good nutrition can mean to them and how they can use the foods available to them to be well nourished.

An inspiring example of what can be accomplished with creative thinking and lavish amounts of hard work is found in Puerto Rico.

THE DONA ELENA PROJECT IN PUERTO RICO

In an isolated mountain community in Puerto Rico, the long-term study known as the Dona Elena Project was conducted. Its objective was to help the families in the community improve their nutrition and other conditions of home and community living.

This project had its origin in a talk the late Dr. Lydia J. Roberts, distinguished Professor of Home Economics at the University of Chicago, had with Mr. Luis Munoz, who was then the governor of Puerto Rico. Some years ago after retiring from the University of Chicago, Dr. Roberts moved to San Juan and became affiliated with the School of Home Economics at the University of Puerto Rico.

The governor had expressed his gratification at the improvement in the general economy of the island under the industrialization program, but he voiced his concern for the rural families in remote areas. Dr. Roberts told the governor of a "pipe dream" she had long had—to select a remote rural community of some 100 or so families, make a detailed study of all aspects of living conditions and, on the basis of the findings, have all governmental agencies concerned plan and carry out a program designed to raise the standard of living in these families.

This idea was offered not as a solution to the problem, but as an approach which might point the way to procedures that could help solve the problem in this and similar communities. The governor was enthusiastic; funds were made available, and the project was on.

The community chosen was Dona Elena Alto, which consisted of some 100 homes in a mountainous section in a tobacco-growing area about two hours from San Juan. The last five miles to reach Dona Elena had to be completed by jeep, on foot, or on a horse.

For practical reasons, the program was started as a nutrition project, letting other aspects enter in as the need should arise. The program was centered around the school and the school lunch program, and the growth and physical status of the children were used as one index of results. All families in the area were, however, included in the educational program. A similar community just over the mountain ridge from Dona Elena was used as the control.

What was done: community and individual action for more vegetable gardens; more fruit trees, more chickens, cows, and pigs; instruction in meal planning and better breakfasts; improved sanitation, housing, water supply, and roads.

Some of the results: the majority of the children showed improved growth by several standards, for example by amounts equal to one-fourth to one-third of a year's normal increment for both weight and height. Improvement in family meals was most apparent in breakfasts. At the start of the project only six families had any vegetable gardens, and in five years fifty families had gardens. During the five-year program, about two-thirds of the families began raising chickens, and the flocks were a good breed for egg production.

Anyone familiar with food preferences in Puerto Rico and other areas south of the U.S. is well aware of the frequent use of beans and rice in the diet. All too often there is a tendency to overlook the nutritive strengths of such staple items.

THE MERITS OF PLANT PROTEINS

"Beans and rice, please." Such an order is appropriate for the visitor to Puerto Rico who wishes to eat the foods common to the area. Beans and rice is certainly a common and preferred dish not only in Puerto Rico, but also in many other parts of the world—Central America, and parts of Latin America and Asia, to say nothing of Louisiana and a few other southern states in the U.S.

Nutritionally beans and rice make good sense because their protein tends to supplement each other in nutritional quality. The protein of rice is slightly superior nutritionally to the proteins of the other common cereals such as corn and wheat, though rice is a little lower in total protein—7 to 8 percent compared with 9 to 12 percent in the raw or dry grains. The protein of legumes (beans and peas are legumes) is better nutritionally than the protein in cereals because of the mixture of amino acids and the larger quantity of protein (20 to 23% in the dry bean).

In the Department of Biochemistry and Nutrition of the Medical School at the University of Puerto Rico, Professor Jose A. Gayco and Dr. C. F. Asenjo studied the nutritional qualities, particularly the quality of the protein, of different legumes consumed in the Caribbean. There are good legumes and bad ones, though perhaps it is better to say there are good legumes and better ones. At the top of their list is the chick pea and the soybean, at the bottom are native red beans and red kidney beans, and intermediate in nutritional value are California chick peas, pigeon peas, and lima beans.

Nutritional quality is usually evaluated by feeding the material as the only source of protein at a definite level in the diet of a growing animal, usually the young rat, and measuring the growth of the animal. Thus we can compare the weight gain of the animal over a test period of two or three weeks with the amount of protein eaten. The reference standard is usually taken to be the protein of dried whole egg or of milk protein (casein).

Drs. Gayco and Asenjo found legumes varied by almost 100 percent in their protein quality. These findings have great practical value in improving the nutrition of people who depend on beans and rice as their main nutriment day after day, year after year. Thus, a way to improve "beans and rice" nutritionally is to say "chick peas, beans and rice, please!" But of course, if we want to do the best job nutritionally, put a little meat or fish in with the rice dish and have some fruit for dessert.

The protein content of beans and rice is vital in helping innumerable people around the world avoid a condition that has created world-wide concern. If you read the newspapers and current magazines very much, you have probably bumped headlong into a word with almost more consonants than you can count. It seems that someone must surely have made a typographical error and either slipped in some extra consonants or left out a vowel or two. The name of this seemingly unpronounceable nutritional deficiency condition is kwashiorkor.

KWASHIORKOR—A CHILD-CENTERED CONCERN

Kwashiorkor doesn't even sound like a word in our language. In fact, it came into the English language only recently from Africa, one of the regions where this condition is found all too often in young children. However, Africa is not the only continent where children develop kwashiorkor because of poor diets. This has been a major problem in some areas of Central and South America and also in India. It may come as a shock to our well- if not over-fed selves that this nutritional deficiency condition has even been found in the United States. The actual cause of kwashiorkor is lack of adequate protein in the diet. In our country, we rely heavily on meat for protein, but meat is terrifically expensive and also not very available in some countries. The necessary protein can also be obtained from milk and dairy products, but often in countries where kwashiorkor is a serious problem, there is no refrigeration and pasteurized milk is not easily obtained. As long as babies are nursed by their mothers, they are getting the protein they need to avoid kwashiorkor. The problem develops when young children are weaned. They often no longer have milk given to them to drink, and meats are too difficult for young children to chew; besides meat is given to them too rarely to provide the amount of protein their growing bodies must have for good health.

Their resistance to infection is poor so they easily become ill. They may also acquire intestinal parasites because of their difficult living conditions. Sickness and parasites cause a still greater need for protein, and the young children between the ages of one and four or five gradually develop kwashiorkor. This disease is truly pathetic to see.

The children with kwashiorkor may have very bloated-looking bodies, or they may be reduced to living skeletons. Their skin will develop dark splotches and will become dry and scaly, and their hair may begin to show a reddish streak or flag where it grows out from the scalp. Although kwashiorkor can be prevented with diets adequate in protein, youngsters with kwashiorkor die each year because they are not adequately fed.

Fortunately, some of the afflicted children are taken to hospitals where they are treated and fed back to health, but the problem could have been avoided if parents could be educated to feed milk and meat or eggs to their children when they are no longer receiving mother's milk.

There is a great need for nutrition education all around the world if kwashiorkor and other nutritional deficiency conditions are to become a matter of historical record rather than a living fact. You can be sure that you and your family have the necessary protein if you drink milk at least twice a day (children drink up to a quart of milk daily), and if you also serve meat, eggs, or cheese daily. Of course, baked beans, pinto beans, refried beans, beans and rice, and split pea soup are other good protein sources to serve.

Much research on kwashiorkor has been done in Guatemala City at the Institute of Nutrition of Central America and Panama, commonly referred to as INCAP.

INCAPARINA

In Guatemala, the staple food is corn, and only small amounts of animal protein are eaten. Adults can exist on this monotonous diet, but post-weanling children cannot. The stress placed upon the human from parasitosis and other infectious diseases, in addition to lack of sufficient, nutritionally-adequate food, particularly protein, results in the child developing kwashiorkor, a common and frequently fatal disease, and the adult becoming anemic, weak, and nonproductive.

At INCAP Dr. Nevin S. Scrimshaw and his co-workers developed a food acceptable to many in Central America, a food adequate in quality protein and low enough in cost so it can be procured by those who need it. It will prevent and treat kwashiorkor. It is called "Incaparina" and consists of corn, cottonseed meal, sorghum, and a small amount of yeast, plus added vitamin A, lysine and calcium. It has the odor of corn, and this helps establish it as an acceptable food.

Another example of improving the nutritive quality of a popular food, which by itself is grossly inadequate, comes from our experience in Latin America. In Colombia, protein-calorie malnutrition (kwashiorkor specifically) is as rampant in various groups of children as it is in Guatemala. Panella, an unrefined type of sugar that is sold in block form (resembling old-fashioned dark laundry soap), is consumed as such, or mixed with water and fed to the children. For many individuals, it constitutes the main source of calories. Even when milk may occasionally be added to the sugar mixture, it is often diluted to such an extent that there is not sufficient protein for the growth and well-being of the child.

Dr. J. J. Vitale, when he was with Harvard's Department of Nutrition, working in Cali, and Dr. O. Phillips, Director of the Institute of Technical Research in Bogota, collaborated on a program to develop a food that looks and tastes like Panella, but which contains a significant amount of a concentrated soy protein extract. Preliminary animal studies and a few metabolic studies with infants and children attested to the improved nutritive qualities of this Panella-like product. Acceptance by both mother and child has been gratifying.

Both of these new products, Incaparina and the soy protein Panella, were modifications of indigenous foods, modifications to improve the diet and combat a serious and common problem in public health due to lack of protein.

When a new product is introduced, careful instruction must be given to the user or the new product may actually be used in such a way as to be harmful. For example, proprietary baby food and dried skim milk have become commonplace in the feeding of infants in many underdeveloped countries. However, the importance of following directions in the preparation of the formula has not always been made sufficiently clear to the women. Mothers in these areas frequently dilute the dried products to less than one-fourth of the amount recommended and add cassava flour to a small amount of formula or dried skim milk, causing it to appear white and therefore acceptable to them, but actually of poor nutritive quality.

The spread of nutrition information has been accomplished in many remote parts of the world. Although the information may be quite sketchy and not too well understood, at least the seed of nutrition knowledge has reached impressive numbers of people.

NUTRITION "KNOWLEDGE" IN A PERUVIAN VILLAGE

You might be interested in some observations made by Dr. Edwin Wellin, a social anthropologist formerly associated with Harvard's Department of Nutrition, who investigated feeding practices in a Peruvian village. He found mothers know about orange juice and vitamins. They had heard about them in the health centers and from city relatives.

Orange and other citrus juice is endorsed by all health workers in Peru. It is referred to by the Peruvian mother as "something recommended by doctors." However, most mothers in this village still believe no child should be given orange juice while consuming only milk. They believe the child must acquire resistance to solid foods before receiving orange juice, and hence they do not use orange juice as a supplement to milk feeding.

These mothers were not aware that more than one vitamin exists, but they did believe that the vitamin existed in other foods, particularly meat and fish. They make their own interpretation of the nutrition information given to them. They believe that the vitamin is a "strong substance," which imparts strength and vigor to foods, but they also believe that pregnant women and children should not have "strong food." Therefore, vitamin-laden foods are too strong for the infants, children, and pregnant women, and so the very people who need the nutrients of citrus fruit, meat, and fish the most are deprived of them.

In these situations the small amount of nutrition information taught was redefined by the subjects and in the process, vitamins, orange juice, and protein foods were interpreted by the Peruvians to be unsuitable for pregnancy, infancy, and childhood.

Nutrition problems in developing countries cannot be solved by the importation or cultivation of foods strange to the people, without considerable planning. A vigorous nutrition education campaign is an integral part of instituting any change in the diet. This campaign must be carried on at all socioeconomic and political levels. Any sound nutritional program must include foods indigenous to the country and available at a cost commensurate with the economic status of the people in need. It must include repeated demonstrations of the need and the use of the food to the person responsible for its usage. Teaching methods must involve the grass roots and must be practical and acceptable.

And the health problems created by inadequate diets are not limited to the Western Hemisphere. The following description of nutrition problems can be applied to practically any area where living conditions and income are substandard.

THE PRICE OF BEING A "HAVE-NOT"

Starvation haunts the "have-not" nations of the world, and poses a critical threat to human welfare and world peace. Pictures of gaunt people are a vivid reminder that right now most of the millions of people who live in Asia, Africa, Central and South America are seriously underfed.

In those areas people have a daily average of 1,000 fewer calories than we do, less than half as much protein, and only ⅕ as much of valuable animal protein. Why? Largely because of primitive agricultural practices, aggravaged by poor food habits due to misery, ignorance, and taboos.

At its worst, this protein-calorie malnutrition causes two diseases—kwashiorkor and marasmus—which produce severe emaciation in infants and young children. Still, dramatic recovery can be achieved with adequate diet therapy; so feeding these starving youngsters becomes both urgent and rewarding.

Chronic malnutrition, although not always life-threatening, is responsible for many diseases. Blindness afflicts thousands; yet this could easily be prevented in many instances if daily meals contained enough vitamin A. Beriberi is widespread, but this, too, could be eliminated if milled rice were enriched with thiamin (one of the B vitamins). Other nutritional deficiencies cause pellagra and anemias, and diarrhea is common as a result of inadequate food and poor sanitation.

Less severe malnutrition leads to other complications. In children, growth is greatly retarded; this helps explain the small stature of people in the under-developed countries. In adults, hunger diminishes vigor and ambition, and work capacity is reduced. The sad result is decreased food production, so hunger goes on and on in a self-perpetuating cycle.

An added complication is the interrelationship between malnutrition and infection. In a review of this whole subject, Dr. Nevin S. Scrimshaw and Dr. Moises Behar of Guatemala emphasize that infection can precipitate nutritional disease. Furthermore, malnutrition decreases resistance to infection and increases mortality. For instance, in the single period 1959–60, mortality from measles was 180 times higher in Mexico, 189 times higher in Guatemala, and 418 times higher in Ecuador than in the United States. Surveys by other workers have established that in the under-developed countries malnutrition alone causes as much as ⅓ of the deaths of young children, and it contributes to deaths from other causes.

On the other hand, proper nutrition lessens both the risk and the severity of infection and reduces mortality. One group of mothers and children under age five showed spectacular improvement in health only because they had received an extra 15 grams of animal protein (about a half-ounce) and 450 calories five days each week for five years.

Therein lies the hope and the goal for the future. It is encouraging to remember that in our United States, scurvy, rickets, pellagra, and beriberi were common up to 50 years ago, and there were many more deaths then than now from diarrhea and the ordinary children's diseases. The fact that this pattern could be altered so dramatically in a relatively short time shows what can be done, and what now must be done in other parts of the world. As malnutrition is decreased, health and well-being will increase and with that comes happiness and world peace.

Wars in the past have provided unfortunate illustrations of nutritional deficiencies, and one of these can be found in Central Europe today.

RICKETS—A REMINDER OF WORLD WAR I

Bowed legs, goiter, and obesity are nutritional problems that can be noted in people in their 60's by the trained observer in Central Europe. The age is important, for people in their 60's would have been children during the first World War. At that time there was no synthetic vitamin D, and most people were dependent on cod liver oil from Norway for that vitamin. These supplies were stopped, so children particularly in Central Europe had little chance of receiving adequate amounts of vitamin D. Thus there was poor and slow calcification of bones, with the result that the long bones of the leg were weak and bowed under the strain of learning to walk and the running and jumping of childhood.

Today we are not dependent on fish liver oils for vitamin D because it now can be made synthetically at a price much cheaper than fish liver oil. Shortly after synthetic vitamin D became available, it frequently was added to milk, particularly evaporated milk which was and still is the backbone of many infant feeding formulas. For many years, vitamin D has been added in small amounts to the diet to prevent rickets. Consequently, rickets, of which bowed legs is one of the physical signs, has practically disappeared from the United States and from many other countries where it once was prevalent.

Vitamin D is also made by our skin through the action of the ultraviolet rays of the sun. It is called the "sunshine vitamin" because of this formation in the body. Strangely, bowed legs and other manifestations of rickets have frequently been present in sunny lands that have the custom of keeping infants and children either out of the sun or covering them well when they are outside.

Certainly there is ample evidence that nutrition problems have existed around the world in the past, and there is every indication that these problems will become intensifed as the world's population grows.

NUTRITION IN PERSPECTIVE

Count one. In that moment, three babies were born somewhere in the world.

Now count to seven. In that brief time, a baby was born somewhere in the United States.

At this rate, in roughly ninety years, the population of the world will have increased to seven billion! Here in the United States there will be 600 million people. That is more than the whole world's population in 1700 and about three times the present population of the United States.

What tons of milk and meat, potatoes and tomatoes, bread and butter will be required to feed such vast number! Will there be enough? The tremendous strides of the past 100 years give us hope for the next century, if we continue to apply our knowledge with intelligence and understanding of the vast problems involved.

In President Lincoln's time, six million farm workers were needed to provide the food for 30 million Americans. Today each farmer can produce enough for 26 individuals, representing more than a five-fold increase in farming efficiency.

Engineers have helped through constructing dams and irrigation systems. Experts in breeding have done wonders developing new crop strains that will withstand different kinds of soil, weather, and pests. Techniques of plowing, fertilizing, and planting have advanced. Inventors and manufacturers have constantly improved farming machinery. Good transportation has made it possible for fresh food to travel quickly and in good condition from farm to store to home.

Success has also depended on destruction of the insects, diseases, and weeds which can cause huge losses in crop yield and in farmers' incomes. Statistics show that without pesticides and chemicals, it would not be possible to achieve the impressive production records of recent years. Of course, these chemicals must be carefully handled. Government workers and food processors are continually working to define and maintain appropriate procedures for and levels of use of chemicals to optimize crop production without causing deleterious effects on humans.

But despite the many advances that have been made, there is no surplus of food in the world today. There is a great hunger belt in today's world that extends from Asia across Africa to South America. In this region, millions of people are slowly starving to death.

The United States must continue not only to feed her increasing population, but also to free others from hunger. If we intensify our own production and distribute it wisely, and if we share with less favored nations the knowledge and skills we have developed, we can make a tremendous contribution to human welfare.

One outstanding example of international efforts to improve nutrition can be seen in the Philippines at the International Rice Institute where agricultural scientists have been working on many approaches to improving the nutrition of the large rice-eating population of the world. New varieties of rice have been developed there. These varieties have been bred to produce a larger yield of rice per acre and to be more resistant to various pests that attack the rice plants and reduce the yield. Insecticides and fertilizers to improve the yield have been carefully researched.

The problems were many. For example, one strain of rice was developed that had a very large yield of rice, but the head of the plant was then so heavy that the stalk could no longer hold it up, and the rice fell over into the paddy and rotted. Finally, a stronger stalk was bred and the heavy yield of rice could then be supported above the water.

Of course, such information is of little value unless it can be put to use by the rice growers in the rice-eating lands. To solve this, the Rice Institute trains representatives from the various countries to go back to their own countries and work with the local farmers. This work is paying dividends in increased rice production to help feed a growing population.

Perhaps the complexity of the problems being attacked by the Rice Institute and other agencies coping directly with the food supply problem can be better understood by looking at India's problems, for surely no other country faces more serious food shortages than that heavily populated country.

INDIA'S FOOD PROBLEM

Press reports continually emphasize the seriousness of India's food problem. There clearly is not enough food to fill all stomachs with enough energy to keep body and soul together, to say nothing about energy for many of its people to work at maximum efficiency.

The basic food in much of India is wheat; in other parts of India it is rice and millet. Pulses (edible plant seeds) are also consumed, but in highly varying amounts, and usually at relatively low levels. While these three cereals are good sources of energy when consumed in sufficient amounts, their protein is inadequate because the level of lysine, an essential constituent of nutritionally complete protein, is inadequate. However, the protein value of these cereals can be made complete either by adding a small amount of lysine to enrich the cereals or by including a little meat or other animal protein in the diet to provide the missing lysine.

Lack of enough protein in the diet, or protein of poor nutritional quality gives rise to kwashiorkor. The poor development of muscles, lack of resistance to infectious diseases, lethargy, and other symptoms of protein deficiency are accentuated when the diet is also low in total calories, as is too often the case.

Basically two steps are needed to solve India's food and nutritional status problems: (1) produce or import more of the staple foods, that is, wheat, rice, and millet to provide more calories and more protein, and (2) improve the nutritional quality of the proteins of the diet.

The first step, that of producing or importing more cereal grains is a problem of agriculture and economics, but it is easier to produce more of a crop one is accustomed to eating than it is to attempt to develop other foods. Also the yield of food energy and protein per acre of land is high in cereal production as compared with raising animal foods and most other acceptable vegetable foods.

Production and distribution problems revolve around such facts as: the arable land in Japan produces three to four times as much food per acre as does land in India; countries needing more food cannot afford to buy it; and surpluses are really comparatively small in terms of having much effect on the huge calorie deficit of the world's hungry millions. To use surpluses to help the promotion of economic and social development, to aid in the leveling out of inequalities, and to make a large and long-term effort to attack malnutrition in the world are monumental tasks.

The second step in meeting India's (and the world's) food crisis is improving the protein quality of the diet. One way of doing this is to produce, import, and consume more meat, fish, eggs, milk, and pulses. The superior protein of these foods, when consumed in sufficient amounts, will improve the lysine-deficient protein of the wheat, rice, and millet. This is an appropriate procedure which may prove to be unrealistic, impractical, and even impossible for a country that is short of food and where agricultural practices are only beginning to be modernized. It takes time to adapt agricultural methods to the production of new crops. These protein foods are much lower in yield of calories per acre of land needed to produce them. One might assume that these foods would be eaten by the people once they were made available, an assumption that unfortunately ignores the fact that food habits ingrained by centuries of tradition and culture are not readily changed. Perhaps a far more practical approach is to improve the nutritional quality of the proteins of cereals by adding lysine. Prior to a few years ago, this would not have been feasible because of the expense of lysine. However, chemists in a few competing world industries have now discovered ways for preparing lysine in large quantity, and the price is economically feasible.

Clearly, plans for feeding the world must take note of the food prejudices and preferences that prevail throughout the world.

ONE MAN'S FOOD IS ANOTHER MAN'S POISON

Illustration of the old saying that "one man's food is another man's poison" is found in the world's history and habits. What is eaten with gusto in one area is refused with horror in another.

Frequently such likes and dislikes interfere with good nutrition. Food prejudices may deprive whole nations of essential nutrients. Gradually some of these preferences will have to be altered if everyone in the world is to be adequately fed. This will take time, for food habits are deeply rooted in the customs and beliefs of a country or group.

Chicken is a good example of contrasting reactions. From Florida to France, from southern-fried chicken to coq au vin, poultry is considered a delicacy. Roast turkey staved off starvation in colonial times and still is a feast for us now. Chicken continues to be both festive dish and vital source of important nutrition throughout China and southeast Asia. Yet the Arabians and some of the Africans do not share this enjoyment at all; they despise chicken and eggs.

Pork is another food that arouses mixed feelings. The ham sandwich is a mainstay of American lunches, but its popularity is by no means worldwide. The Moslems, orthodox Jews, and various sects of the East forbid all eating of pork. Regardless of religion, in Ethiopia no one eats pork; it is scorned by Christians there and other religions alike.

And what about horse meat? For many centuries it was commonly eaten in Europe. The Spaniards even gave it a special name—red deer. To the French it is still a dietary staple, especially for the lower income group. In Asia the Japanese and Chinese eat horse meat without prejudice, but on the other side of the border in Tibet the nomads react as violently as we do against this particular food. Certainly dogs could not be considered food in the United States. In China, however, though dogs are objects of affection, they are also considered worthy of a feast.

In much of India, where the bull and cow are sacred animals, the Hindus will not touch beef or dairy products. Elsewhere in Asia and in some of Africa, there are many who do not think milk is fit for human consumption. We, however, refer to milk as "nature's most nearly perfect food." And we call bread the "staff of life," but half the population of the world prefers rice or corn to wheat.

Some of these differences are slowly vanishing. Developments in agriculture are bringing new methods of cultivation to old lands. Research and education are spreading new ideas. Tastes and taboos shift and change. Pioneers in New England delighted in pemmican (dried meat pounded into shreds, then mixed with fat and berries). The steak that replaces pemmican today may tomorrow be supplanted by space age substitutes. To prepare for the future, we will have to learn to push our prejudices into the past.

You might think that the problems of feeding man on earth are more than enough to keep nutritionists and related scientists scurrying for many, many years, but the unique aspects of feeding man in space have also required considerable attention. Just imagine what you would have to consider if you had the task of providing lunch at an orbiting space station or a picnic on the moon!

FLY ME TO THE MOON (BUT FEED ME ON THE WAY)

Gastronautics is a term that aptly covers the problems of developing adequate foods for man in space. As we have watched the various space expeditions, we have gradually learned more about the nutrition component of the space program. However, these probes appear still in their infancy compared with the possible journeys far beyond the moon. Suppose you had to plan the food, oxygen, and water needs for a four-man crew for a year's journey into outer space. If you over-estimate energy needs by as little as 300 calories per day, you can cause the launching weight to be between 600 and 800 pounds greater than is necessary. And what is worse, if you under-estimate by 300 calories per man per day, not only will they lose weight, but oxygen and water will be exhausted before the mission is completed. Dr. Doris Calloway, Professor of Nutrition at the University of California at Berkeley and a leading researcher in this area of nutrition, has calculated that if you underestimate by 300 calories per day, the oxygen planned for a trip of 14 days will last only 12½ days.

A little mistake in the grocery order cannot be solved by a fast trip to the local supermarket or a handy freezer. It is tricky business to plan meals for a space trip. Food has to be light, compact and low in residue, but tasty, easy to eat, and require a minimum of preparation in the space ship. The menus now are selected to satisfy the food preferences of the astronauts, for it has been a problem to tempt the palate enough to get these voyagers to eat the amount they need for maintenance. Part of the success of the mission is based on the amount of food consumed and the nutritional status of each astronaut upon his return. Even with this devoted attention, it has been difficult to minimize calcium losses during space travel.

The development of these foods for space has been a major concern for NASA. Various government laboratories and private organizations have been involved cooperatively in devising suitable space fare. The first food items were developed by the Air Force for high altitude flights. These foods were the consistency of junior baby foods and were packaged in toothpaste-type tubes with a special feeding tube attached. Later some chewy foods such as malted milk balls and fruit-flavored candy-wafers were included. Specifications for developing new foods included a tolerance of temperatures of 110°F, 100 percent relative humidity, and no crumbling or breakup at 15 G's shock. Under these restrictions, the development of freeze-dried foods was a tremendous breakthrough. Coatings of edible films were a solution to the crumb problem for food packaged in bite-size pieces.

Everyone associated with the manned flight program realized the need for exercise for the astronauts, but ways of achieving it are not easy. Unfortunately exercise just cannot be compressed into cubes, dried, and put into packages for easy consumption. Considerable work has gone into exploring the problems of keeping fit during long periods of relative inactivity and weightlessness, and it appears that there is still much to do. Meantime, all this work and worry provides more proof that activity cannot be taken for granted. It is no less important for us than for the astronauts, though we are not on our way to the moon. And it is far easier for us than for the astronauts because we have plenty of room and opportunity.

Whether exploring in space or plodding along on earth, each one of us needs to figure out the best activity for getting our muscles into shape and keeping them that way. Exercise every day to be fit now and to keep old age at bay.

9

A COOK'S TOUR OF NUTRITION

We have looked at weight control problems, diets for various health conditions, food facts, world nutrition problems, sensible and healthful marketing, and various other aspects of nutrition in this book. As a bit of a bonus to you in your quest for nutrition information, we have decided to write this final chapter as an overall review of nutrition, to summarize the nutrients—what they are, what they do, and what to eat to obtain them.

To most of us, food has meaning in a psychological, physiological, and social sense. Close your eyes and think about the last holiday dinner. Did you remember special foods for the occasion and a table that almost sagged from the weight of the fare? These warm thoughts of food and the comfort it brings are what we call the psychological meaning of food. Certainly that is important to all of us.

Let's think now about what you would do if a good friend stopped by to visit you. It is almost a sure bet that you would offer him or her something to eat or drink. In our culture, our first thoughts of friendship and hospitality concern what food to serve for the occasion. Food, partly because of its psychological and physiological values to us, is almost always a part of any social gathering.

The physiological value of food is clear to us all. We all know that a person will die eventually if he does not have food to eat. However, it is remarkable how long some people have managed to live during a fast. A Frenchman named Merlatte successfully went without food for 50 days, and Terence MacSwiney, Irish Mayor of Cork, fasted for 74 days before dying in a coma as a result of a hunger strike. Then there is the story of two people who were finally rescued after a 48-day ordeal following the crash of their plane in the Yukon. These two people survived on a total of two cans of sardines, two cans of fruit cocktail, and water from the snow. It was the water that provided the key to their survival, for water is more critical to the body than food. Water is the medium for removing waste materials and is essential for all the life processes carried on in the cells. Water is constantly lost by evaporation through the skin (in perspiration), through the lungs (in breathing), and by excretion through the intestinal tract and the kidneys. Adults cannot live much more than one week without water.

However, even with all the water they needed, it seems impossible that these people could have survived almost seven weeks on a total of approximately 2,100 calories. They were fortunate in that neither of them had serious injuries which would have added to their nutritional needs. They were both in good health at the time of the crash, again avoiding the complication of unusual nutritional requirements. In a sense, they were lucky to have the supplies needed to keep warm, to have the psychological will to survive, and to be able to remain very inactive, thus reducing caloric needs.

It is clear from the experience of these two in the Yukon that water is definitely an essential nutrient for survival. However, there are many other substances needed by the body for growth, maintenance, and good health. We all need energy for a variety of purposes. The most obvious one is for moving the body, either to do work or to play. We also need energy for carrying on all the essential activities of the body even while we are asleep. When you stop to think about it, you realize that the heart must beat continually, breathing is a continuous process requiring energy, and several other ongoing operations of the body could also be cited that dictate a constant need for energy just to live. We also need to have energy to utilize the food we have eaten for energy, just another aspect of the cycle on which we operate. Energy is available from three different types of nutrients: carbohydrates, fats, and proteins.

CARBOHYDRATES

At one time there was almost a halo around foods that gave you energy. Candy frequently was advertised as the quick energy food. With American preoccupation with weight control, the merits of carbohydrates as sources of energy have been relegated to the background in advertisements lately.

Carbohydrates deserve a better reputation than they have been awarded in the past several decades. With the exception of fiber, carbohydrates are a practical and easily utilized source of energy. All carbohydrates are organic materials made of carbon, hydrogen, and oxygen. The simple carbohydrates are quickly absorbed and available to maintain the blood sugar, a factor that helps us feel energetic. This is why a product containing sugar gives us a quick lift when we eat it. Even food containing brown sugar or honey will provide energy to the body quite rapidly.

All the different types of sugar-containing foods, including candy, syrups (corn and table), jellies and jams, honey, and sugars (granulated, powdered, maple, and brown), are easy-to-use sources of calories for energy. In addition, there are more complex carbohydrates that are used more slowly, thus making additional energy available after the calories from the sugars have already been used. All types of starches are examples of these complex carbohydrates. These are found in bread, cereals, legumes (beans and peas), corn, and potatoes.

Fiber is an unusual example of complex carbohydrates, and performs a unique function in the body. Humans are not equipped with the enzyme needed to break it down so that energy can be procured. Instead, fiber remains essentially unchanged as it moves through the digestive tract. The coarse texture of fiber is useful because it helps to move food materials along the tract and facilitates excretion of waste.

FATS

Fats frequently are described as a concentrated source of energy. Indeed, this is an accurate analysis, for a gram of fat provides nine calories to the body compared with only four calories per gram from either carbohydrates or proteins. A calorie (also called a kilocalorie) is defined here as the amount of heat needed to raise one kilogram (roughly one quart) of water 1° centigrade. Not only are pure fats rich sources of calories because of the energy released when they are metabolized in the body, but they are quite concentrated in many of the foods rich in fats so that you do not need to eat a large volume of fat in order to get a fairly large number of calories for energy. The person with a relatively small capacity for food and a large need for calories may appreciate this concentrated source of calories. To people with a weight problem, this characteristic of fats such as butter does not hold great fascination.

In addition to its value as a source of calories, fat is needed in the body to supply an essential fatty acid known as linoleic acid, and also to carry the fat-soluble vitamins, A, D, E, and K, into the body. Linoleic acid, like all other fat molecules, is made up of carbon, hydrogen, and oxygen, thus is classified as an organic compound. However, unlike many of the fatty acids, linoleic acid does not contain all of the hydrogen it is capable of holding. It is classified as a polyunsaturated fatty acid, and its formula cannot be created by our bodies from any other type of fat molecule. Yet, this particular substance is needed for health of the skin. Without linoleic acid, infants will develop a very dry and scaly skin.

Remember that fat is needed in the diet to serve as a carrier of these four essential nutrients, the fat-soluble vitamins. These days we hear fat maligned so often that it is easy to forget that fat does perform these other functions in addition to providing calories for energy.

Fats are found in many foods, sometimes as visible fats and sometimes seemingly invisible. It is obvious that butter and margarine are fats, and one can easily determine how much is being spread on a piece of bread. Other visible fats include fat on a cut of meat, cream, whipped cream, and other foods that are recognized as being high in fat content. However, some people are less aware of fat contained in salad dressings, well marbled meats such as high quality beef and pork, and in avocados and nuts. All of these foods are good sources of fat. And one certainly should not overlook pastries and fried foods, including onion rings, French fries, and potato chips!

This table will give you a picture of some of the contributions of various animal products.

FAT CONTENT OF SELECTED ANIMAL PRODUCTS

Food	% Fat	Food	% Fat
Lard	99.0	Ice cream	12.0
Butter	86.0	Veal	6–15
Bacon	72.0	Eggs	10.0
Whipping cream	36.0	Chicken	5.0
Cream cheese	35.0	Fish	0.1–10.0
Ham, pork	25.0	Whole milk	3.5–4.0
Lamb	16–20	Yogurt	2.0
Beef	10–16	Cottage cheese	0.5
Coffee cream	16.0	Skim milk	0.1

PROTEIN

Proteins, like carbohydrates and fats, are organic compounds found in foods, but they contain nitrogen as well as carbon, hydrogen, and oxygen. The significance of protein as a nutrient is indicated by its name; protein comes from a Greek word meaning first. Protein is of first importance because it is the chief constituent of all body tissues. It is essential to make new cells and to repair old ones. Without protein, children's growth will be stunted, and adults will waste away. Protein is also essential for antibody formation. It is needed for hormones and enzymes. Although it is an expensive use of protein, the body can also use it for energy if necessary.

Proteins are made up of building blocks called amino acids. Various amino acids are combined in all sorts of ways to make the many different proteins found in plants and animals. When we eat proteins, the body breaks down the protein molecules into the individual amino acids and then uses these to make the proteins specifically needed. Some of the amino acids can be changed into other amino acids that may be needed to construct a particular protein in the body. If an amino acid can be made from another one in the body, the amino acid is said to be non-essential. There are eight amino acids that are needed to make proteins for the human body, but which the body itself cannot make.

These eight amino acids must be obtained from the foods we eat; they are called essential amino acids.

With the exception of gelatin, the proteins from animal foods contain all the essential amino acids plus many of the non-essential amino acids. These are called complete proteins. Cereals and legumes are also valuable sources of protein in the diet, although the proteins they contain may be lacking one or more of the essential amino acids. These incomplete plant proteins are important to help meet the body's need for protein without the high cost involved when all the protein is provided from animal sources. By using both animal and vegetable proteins, it is possible to be well nourished and to moderate the cost of protein. In summary, animal protein sources include milk, cheese, eggs, poultry, fish, beef, lamb, pork, and other types of meats. Dried beans (kidney, soy, navy, pinto, lima, etc.), black-eyed peas, split peas, nuts, rice, and other cereals and breads are good vegetable protein sources.

The shortage of protein which the consumer can afford is perhaps the most critical aspect of meeting the world's nutrition problems. In many countries of the world animal protein is scarce and fearfully expensive. Millions have to be without it, especially in China and the Far East, Africa, Asia, and some of South America. Large segments of the population suffer, particularly those who are most in need of protein: infants and young children, and the women who bear and nurse them.

Although the usual dietary pattern provides protein from both animal and plant sources, it is possible to obtain protein from a wide variety of vegetable sources and thus get all of the essential amino acids, but it is very difficult to be sure that an appropriate balance of amino acids has been incorporated in the diet. If milk, cheese, or eggs can be included, the essential amino acids required for good health will be insured.

MINERALS

Perhaps you have seen the sobering analysis of the value of the human body in terms of the structural materials represented. It really is a bit deflating to consider that even with the inflation of today, the components of our bodies add up to significantly less than a five dollar bill! Fortunately, humans are an outstanding example of the value of the whole being far greater than the numerical sum of its parts. But enough of the philosophizing. Let's turn our attention to the minerals that make up the human body.

There are seven minerals known as macronutrients because they are essential for human nutrition and comprise 0.05 percent or more of the body's total weight. In descending order of quantity in the body, they are calcium (1.5 to 2.2% of body weight), followed by phosphorus, potassium, sulphur, sodium, chlorine, and magnesium. The essential micronutrients range in quantity from 0.004 percent of the body weight for iron down to only 0.00004 percent for iodide. The essential micronutrients are iron, zinc, selenium, manganese, copper, iodide, molybdenum, cobalt, vanadium, barium, fluoride, bromide, strontium, chromium, tin, and no doubt others yet to be found.

Calcium, the most abundant of the body's minerals, performs such important jobs as helping to make bones and teeth hard, regulating the heart beat, and even clotting the blood. For the best growth possible, calcium must be available in adequate quantities all through childhood. All through life, calcium protects the integrity of bones and teeth by making them strong. This is important in preventing broken bones and lost teeth. Of course, calcium is available in several different foods, with milk being the outstanding source. Cheese of all types also adds to the intake of calcium, as do sardines and other fish containing edible bones, broccoli, kale, and other greens. Spinach and rhubarb contain oxalic acid which causes some formation of an insoluble calcium salt, thus slightly reducing the absorption of calcium. However, this is not a problem of any consequence in the quantities these foods are found in the diet.

Although iron is classified as a micronutrient on the basis of its total weight in the body, it clearly is one of the more important minerals. In fact, this is one mineral that deserves much more attention in people's diets. According to recent nationwide information, iron is inadequate in the diets of many girls and women. Recently there have been extensive advertising campaigns and reasonably extensive coverage of this nutrition inadequacy by several periodicals. There is good reason to be concerned about this mineral.

Iron is required to make a compound called hemoglobin, which is the oxygen-carrying compound in the blood. When adequate iron is available, the hemoglobin level in the blood will be within the normal range (approximately 13 grams per 100 milliliters of blood for women, and 14 to 15 for men). If the iron is not available, the hemoglobin level in the blood decreases, with the result that less oxygen is transported to the various tissues of the body. This drop in hemoglobin level causes a constant feeling of fatigue, and every movement becomes an effort. Obviously, a person who is deficient in iron will not be very productive. Just living seems to become almost too much effort. Persons with a low hemoglobin level have iron-deficiency anemia. One commercial company has given this type of anemia the colorfully appropriate name of "tired blood."

You might think that you would know immediately if you were anemic, yet this condition may creep up so gradually that a person is unaware of the very slow development of lethargy and general fatigue. It is important to be aware of your iron intake throughout your life, but there are certain times in life when an iron-deficiency condition is more likely to develop. Whenever a child is growing very rapidly, it is necessary to pay particular attention to the hemoglobin level and be certain that he is getting enough iron. Young women in their child-bearing years also need to be certain that they are eating enough foods rich in iron.

It takes some good planning to be certain that you are eating enough iron in your diet each day. You could, of course, elect to eat a couple of slices of liver every day to supply your body's need for iron, but most people would find this a bit monotonous. All meats are reasonably good sources, although liver and heart are particularly rich in this mineral. Dried fruits, such as raisins, prunes, peaches, and apricots are concentrated sources of iron. However, you will find that you would need to drink 1¾ cups of prune juice if you are a woman or merely a cup if you are a man in order to provide the day's requirement for iron. Other ways of adding to your iron intake are baked beans, leafy vegetables, lima beans, kidney beans, egg yolks, enriched breads and cereals, and gingerbread. Be sure to include these foods in your diet frequently to avoid the tired feeling that comes when you have an iron deficiency.

One of the important mineral foods in the diet is salt. As it is generally purchased, salt is sodium chloride plus a small amount of potassium iodide. Salt is important in the diet as a means of regulating the osmotic pressure in the body so that the cells will contain a normal level of fluid. In a few instances in very hot regions where people have been doing very hard physical labor and have been sweating profusely, people will lose so much salt through perspiration that they may experience what is commonly called heat prostration. It is to avoid this problem that workers in these stressful conditions used to be given salt pills to replace the excessive losses of sodium and chloride from the body; now we simply recommend a little more salt on food.

The much more usual problem with salt is not a deficiency, but a regular intake that far exceeds what is best for health. It seems to be a favorite ritual of many Americans to invert the salt shaker and observe the salt crystals cascading toward the food. In fact, many people (perhaps you are one of them) habitually salt their food even before they taste it. Although the salt companies may be grateful for your enthusiastic use of salt, your body does not appreciate such treatment. Prolonged high salt intake predisposes some toward developing high blood pressure, a condition which afflicts all too many Americans. You will be doing your body a favor if you reduce your salt intake significantly. It is a reasonable guess that you are consuming ten times as much salt as your body actually needs, and perhaps even as much as 20 times the recommended intake. You can do your body another kindness at the same time if you will form the habit of using only iodized salt. The iodide in iodized salt is essential to health. This mineral is used to make the hormone, thyroxine, which is produced by the thyroid gland to regulate the rate at which your body performs its many autonomic functions. Simply by always using iodized salt, even though you are cutting your salt intake back to lower values, you will get all the iodide you need for making thyroxine. This is your way of protecting against the development of goiter, an enlargement of the thyroid gland.

There is another mineral substance in the body that is chemically related to iodide and which, like iodide, can be added to the diet in small amounts to reap large benefits. This substance is fluoride. Fluoride is a mineral and has been a widely discussed nutrient, one discussed often with more emotion and sentimentality than with actual facts.

FLUORIDE

Prevention of disease is the way of the present and the future. Nowhere is this more promising or important than in the area of nutrition and tooth decay. Adjustment of the fluoride content of community waters (fluoridation) is the most potent prevention today—or in the foreseeable future—for tooth decay. It is not the final answer to the problem, but it will reduce tooth decay by 60 to 70 percent. Perhaps another five percent reduction can be obtained by reducing between-meal eating and by learning to brush teeth every time food is consumed. Neither of these alternative suggestions is very practical, so fluoridation of the water assumes even more importance.

To date, many studies have been done to determine the effectiveness of fluoridation in reducing the incidence of dental caries. If you would like to read about some of these, the National Research Council and the American Dental Association have many publications on this topic. And for an excellent, up-to-date reference, read *The Tooth Robbers: A Pro-Fluoridation Handbook* (George F. Stickley Co., 210 W. Washington Square, Phila., Pa. 19106).

The first interest in fluorides in water arose in a small area of Texas and in Colorado Springs, Colorado, where it was noticed that lifelong residents often had mottled, discolored teeth (Colorado brown stain) that were unusually free of decay. People did not like the appearance of their discolored teeth, but naturally were pleased to have so little problem with the general soundness and health of their teeth. When word of the apparent importance of fluoride in the health of teeth began to spread, attempts to promote sound teeth without staining were tried using lower levels of fluoride than were found in Colorado Springs. The United States Public Health Service used a fluoride level of one part per million (one part fluoride per million parts of water) in its classic study of dental caries in Newburgh, New York in 1945. Kingston children (a city just across the river with unfluoridated water) were the control against which the success of fluoridation was measured. The value of fluoridation for children during their early years was clearly demonstrated, and subsequent studies have shown similar findings.

With today's highly reliable equipment, it is easily possible to accurately control the level of fluoride in the water. The natural fluoride content of the water is determined, and then fluorides are added so that the water supply contains 1 to 1.2 parts per million (ppm). In areas where there is too much fluoride in the water, it is possible to remove some of this mineral to provide water containing the recommended level of fluoride. This is important as an aesthetic aid for children living in areas where the water may contain eight or more parts per million, thus causing discoloration unless the water is defluoridated to the recommended level.

Fluoridation is a money-saver, too. It is estimated that the cost of adding this mineral to water is in the vicinity of 50–75 cents per person per year. Compare this with the cost of having even one filling put in! Of course, it is still necessary to see a dentist for checkups and any needed work, but the number of decayed teeth requiring attention will be greatly reduced.

In addition to the value of fluoridation for the health of the teeth, it is appropriate to mention here that fluoride helps to maintain strong bones in older people, who frequently are beset with the problem of osteoporosis or weakening bones.

If you live in one of the cities where fluoridation is an accomplished fact, you are indeed fortunate. But we have a charge to the rest of the country to take active steps toward making fluoridated water an accepted way of life in the near future. By adjusting the fluoride in the water supply, it is possible to help all children in the city to have better teeth regardless of income, occupation, or family food habits. Fluoride drops, pills, and toothpastes are all better than no fluoride, but these devices are not as effective as fluoridation, and they obviously do not reach many children who deserve fluoridation. Fluoride is important to infants. They will get the fluoride in water, but they certainly will not benefit from fluoridated toothpastes until the teeth have developed enough for brushing. By that age, some of the benefit of fluoridation is already lost.

Perhaps inter-city rivalry can even be used to help speed the cause of fluoridation. Long Beach, California, fluoridates its city water supply. Surely the Mayor and the proud city of Los Angeles cannot long live in the shadow of such modern thinking. It just may be that other communities can find similar motivations.

FAT-SOLUBLE VITAMINS

Vitamins are organic compounds needed in extremely small amounts for the maintenance of life and for growth. These substances frequently are described in such glowing terms that they almost assume super-human importance. In fact, one grandmother when viewing her very energetic granddaughter was heard to muse that "maybe today's children are getting too many vitamins." At any rate, vitamins clearly are essential to everyone. There are several substances that have vitamin activity, and it is common practice to divide them into categories on the basis of their solubility: fat-soluble and water-soluble. The fat-soluble vitamins are vitamin A, D, E, and K.

Vitamin A

How long has it been since you have been to a movie matinee? When we were children, there was something terribly exciting about walking from the brilliant day into the dark cavern of the movie theater. The change was always sudden and impressive. Do you recall with a chuckle the times you almost sat in someone's lap because you couldn't see the seat was occupied? It is customary for people to require a brief period to adjust to changes in light intensity such as this, but some people have a very difficult time adjusting because they are not eating right. Now don't immediately assume that they should have stopped in the lobby for popcorn and candy to improve their vision. The problem goes back a good bit farther than that.

People who adjust very slowly to changes in light intensity are said to have night blindness. This is caused by not having enough vitamin A in the diet. It is easy to eat enough vitamin A from ordinary foods if you follow the Basic Four Food Plan because the fruit and vegetable category stipulates that you should eat a dark green, leafy or a yellow vegetable at least every other day. Simply by eating ⅓ cup of carrots you will get all the vitamin A that you need per day. In the summer you can get enough vitamin A from half a cantaloupe. Greens are outstanding potential sources of vitamin A. One-third cup of spinach or ⅔ cup of kale is enough for the whole day. Or did you know that a mere ⅓ ounce of beef liver supplies all the vitamin A you need? You will notice that both plant and animal sources can be used to provide vitamin A. Actually, the plant sources contain carotene, a substance that can be converted into vitamin A in the body. Liver, egg yolks, butter, milk, and cheese are sources of vitamin A itself.

Lest we leave you with the impression that vitamin A is needed only to prevent night blindness, let's also note that vitamin A helps to keep skin smooth and clear, influences the growth of bones, increases resistance to infection by maintaining the health of the mucous membranes, and prevents a type of blindness known as xerophthalmia.

The recommended amount of vitamin A for adults is 5,000 International Units daily, an amount that is readily supplied simply by judicious selection of vegetables and some animal foods. Remember that massive supplements of this vitamin by taking capsules through self-diagnosis may be harmful if continued for an extended period. Use your food intake to supply vitamin A. It tastes far better this way than in a capsule and is perfectly safe.

Vitamin D

It is difficult to work in any comments about fashions while writing in the field of nutrition, but vitamin D provides an appropriate opportunity. The synonym for vitamin D is the "sunshine vitamin," because vitamin D is formed in the body when the sun's rays hit the skin.

You can easily see that fashions really do influence how much vitamin D you will have available in your body. If you wear clothes that cover practically all of you except your face, you will not form much vitamin D because you will have so little skin exposed. Maybe this vitamin gives a real argument, from a health standpoint, for shorter skirts and bikinis! Even with somewhat less revealing clothes, most of our fashions today promote more production of vitamin D in the skin.

In some countries of the world, clothing styles are considerably different. The classic example of clothing that really interferes with production of vitamin D is worn by women in purdah in some of the Moslem countries. As you know, women in purdah wear garments that cover them completely. There is absolutely no portion of the leg showing, neither is there any arm extending below the sleeve. In fact, the face is even shielded from strangers and the sun by a heavy veil. It is not unusual for girls and women in their child-bearing years to show signs of inadequate vitamin D if they observe the strict customs of purdah. The need for vitamin D is great for girls in their early teens because they are growing rapidly. Women also need this vitamin during their reproductive years if they are to remain healthy and produce healthy, well-formed offspring.

Rickets, a condition caused by a deficiency of vitamin D, may be due either to inadequate diet or a lack of sunshine on the skin. The legs of young children with rickets will begin to bow because the bones are not as hard and rigid as they need to be to support the weight of the body. Calcium, phosphorus, and fluoride all contribute to the strength of bone. People who are normally healthy and who consume sufficient vitamin D will utilize calcium and phosphorus well to form and maintain strong bones and teeth.

An adequate amount of vitamin D is obtained simply by drinking vitamin D-fortified milk daily. Somewhat less vitamin D is needed if you live in a very sunny climate and are outdoors a good deal. As you would guess, the very critical time for vitamin D is during the growing years.

Here we have to caution against the potential hazard of developing hypervitaminosis D if you take pills delivering massive doses of vitamin D. If you count on milk for your source of this vitamin and are not taking vitamin capsules, there is absolutely no reason for you to be concerned about the possibility of having too much vitamin D in your diet. Food sources simply do not supply enough to be harmful; even vitamin D-enriched milk contains a very conservative quantity. To illustrate, a person drinking the unlikely amount of three quarts of milk daily is still getting only three times the recommended daily intake, an amount that clearly presents no health hazard.

The problem stems from the ease with which too much vitamin D can be taken in capsules. It used to be a simple matter for anyone to walk into a drug store and purchase vitamin capsules containing a large quantity of vitamin D. You didn't even have to have a prescription to buy these. All you had to do is pick them off the shelf and pay for them. Then you could take as many as you like each day. Some people are overly concerned about protecting their health with supplements, and these are the persons most likely to take too much vitamin D in pill form. In their concern about providing all the nutrients they need, they may actually harm themselves by taking a level of vitamin D that can damage their bodies.

The exact amount of vitamin D needed to cause hypervitaminosis D is not defined because of the variations in age and body size. Children are far more likely to ingest a harmful dosage over a period of time because of their small body size compared with that of an adult. It does appear that the regular level of vitamin D intake would have to be maintained over a period of time at approximately 12 times the recommended 400 I.U. (4,800 I.U.) before symptoms would begin to develop.

The problems in hypervitaminosis D appear to be related to the excessive deposition of calcium and phosphorus that occurs in the system. The very high levels of vitamin D can increase absorption of these two minerals to the point where a fatal condition may develop from damage to the heart. There has also been some indication that very high levels in lactating women may be transmitted via their milk to young infants and may result in mental retardation.

Vitamins E and K

The other two fat-soluble vitamins have received somewhat less publicity than vitamins A and D. The 1968 revision of the National Research Council's Recommended Daily Dietary Allowances marks the first time vitamin E has been listed. Sometimes you hear vitamin E referred to as the "anti-sterility" vitamin, a name that doubtless has enhanced the sale of this nutrient. The value of this vitamin in the reproductive processes of rats has been demonstrated, but humans have not provided any proof of the value of this vitamin in reproduction. Vitamin E is essential as an anti-oxidant in the body to maintain the activity of other essential and easily oxidized compounds such as vitamin C. The 1973 RDA recommended a reduction in Vitamin E.

Vitamin K, also known as the anti-hemorrhagic vitamin, is essential for the formation of prothrombin, a substance required for the clotting of blood. There is little need to be concerned about the intake of this vitamin because it is synthesized in the intestine.

WATER-SOLUBLE VITAMINS

The water-soluble vitamins are the B vitamins and vitamin C or ascorbic acid. Three of the B vitamins, thiamin, riboflavin, and niacin, are well known. Of lesser fame, but still important are pyridoxine, folacin, vitamin B_{12}, biotin, and pantothenic acid.

The B Vitamins

Thiamin is needed by the body to help release energy from food during metabolism of carbohydrates, fats, and protein. It is also essential in promoting normal appetite and helps in preventing irritability and maintaining a healthy nervous system. A deficiency of thiamin has been a common condition known as beriberi in some parts of the world. If you ever have an opportunity to see someone with this condition, or to even see a movie of a patient with this problem, you will probably promptly resolve to have an adequate amount of thiamin every single day, for this is a truly tragic problem which can easily be avoided simply by eating correctly. Beriberi affects the nerves. One of the symptoms is a feeling of depression, followed by gradual development of a characteristic walk similar to the way you might imagine walking along a very slippery floor covered with small marbles. Persons with advanced beriberi walk very carefully, each foot being lifted abnormally high and painstakingly put down again. An unfortunate complication of beriberi is diarrhea, which only reduces the ability of the body to utilize any thiamin that might be present in the diet. Eventually, severe and untreated beriberi will affect the heartbeat; it is this complication which may lead to the death of the patient. Fortunately, beriberi can be treated and cured by including large amounts of thiamin in the diet. Of course, it can be avoided in the first place if you are simply careful about eating a well-balanced diet regularly.

Pork is a particularly good source of thiamin. In fact, a single 3½-ounce pork chop will provide just over half of the daily requirement of thiamin. Ham, as you would expect, is also an excellent source of this vitamin, and beef and lamb are good sources. Legumes of all types (lima beans, refried beans, baked beans, split pea soup, etc.) are also valuable sources. Enriched cereal products contain significant amounts of thiamin because they are usually eaten regularly during the day. Two servings of meat and four or more servings of whole grain or enriched cereal products will provide the necessary quantity of thiamin.

Riboflavin is another of the B vitamins that is important in the release of energy from the food you eat. Along with the other B vitamins, riboflavin helps to reduce irritability. It also helps to keep the skin, tongue, and mouth healthy. Riboflavin promotes the normal red color of lips and tongue. When riboflavin intake is inadequate, cracks at the corners of the mouth and a purplish red, smooth tongue will be noticed. Dry and scaly skin are other symptoms of ariboflavinosis, the name for the deficiency condition.

You are well on your way toward meeting your riboflavin requirement if you are drinking two glasses of milk each day, and three glasses will supply the entire amount needed. Other good sources are meats of all types, nuts (if you eat them by the cupful), and cheese.

Riboflavin is a somewhat unstable vitamin that needs to be handled with a certain amount of care. This vitamin is water-soluble so it can be lost from meats into the cooking liquid, but more important is the fact that riboflavin is unstable in sunlight. This is of little concern in most food items because we don't ordinarily have a cut of meat sitting in the sunlight nor is milk still delivered to the home, and left on the doorstep along with the morning paper. Most milk is now in opaque cartons to protect it from the light. The harmful rays of the sun cannot go through these packaging materials and the riboflavin will not be lost.

In Chapter 8 we discussed niacin, the B vitamin that is essential if one is to avoid developing pellagra. The activities of *niacin* are somewhat related to those of thiamin and riboflavin. Niacin also functions in releasing energy from food. It is important to the general health of the nervous system, the digestive tract, and the skin, mouth, and tongue.

Rich sources of niacin include meat and poultry, legumes, and enriched or whole grain breads and cereals. Milk and eggs are rich sources of tryptophan, the amino acid that can be converted in the body to the active niacin.

Pyridoxine is a B vitamin found in many foods, but particularly in meats, vegetables, and whole grain cereals. As the study of this B vitamin has progressed, its importance in protein metabolism in the body is becoming more clear. This vitamin is essential for the body to form new amino acids from other compounds. The removal of nitrogen from some amino acids requires pyridoxine. It has also been shown that this vitamin is needed to form a part of the hemoglobin molecule. There is also an indication that this vitamin functions in the utilization of fats and carbohydrates.

Folacin, a B vitamin found abundantly in green, leafy vegetables, is needed in the body for the formation of red blood cells and hemoglobin. In addition, this vitamin is needed to form some of the non-essential amino acids and to produce parts of the nucleic acids, DNA (deoxyribonucleic acid) and RNA (ribonucleic acid). This vitamin is found in broccoli, asparagus, lima beans, strawberries, cantaloupe, liver, kidney, and mushrooms. Since folacin is sensitive to both light and heat, it is wise to be careful with these foods during preparation and to keep cooking time to a minimum for palatability. As we know more of the action of this vitamin and become more aware of possible symptoms of deficiency, more cases of folacin deficiency are being reported. The most readily diagnosed symptom is a megaloblastic anemia characterized by large, immature red blood cells, and sometimes a reduced number of leucocytes.

Vitamin B_{12} is an unusual and rather interesting water-soluble vitamin. Also known as cobalamin, this substance is noteworthy for its effectiveness in treating patients with pernicious anemia. As is true with the other vitamins, vitamin B_{12} is required for normal growth. It is also needed to maintain nervous tissue and to form normal blood. If vitamin B_{12} is inadequate, the red blood cells will be enlarged, as they are in a folacin deficiency. There is absolutely no problem in getting enough vitamin B_{12} in the foods you eat unless you are not eating any animal foods at all. Persons with a vitamin B_{12} deficiency, with the exception of the strictest of vegetarians, have developed the problem as a result of inability to absorb the vitamin from the intestine, not as a result of inadequate diet. Treatment for pernicious anemia generally is by injecting the vitamin, since this avenue avoids the problem of absorption of the needed nutrient.

Biotin is a vitamin that functions in the metabolism of fats, carbohydrates, and some amino acids. Although this vitamin is of interest to researchers, the likelihood of a deficiency is so extremely remote that further consideration of the dietary implications is unnecessary.

Pantothenic acid is one of the B vitamins needed to release energy from food. It is needed to form part of the hemoglobin molecule, to synthesize cholesterol, and to make other molecules. Despite the many ways in which this vitamin functions in the body, deficiency symptoms can usually only be observed by feeding an antagonist that created a deficiency condition. As you might expect, a pantothenic acid deficiency is scarcely even a remote possibility because this substance is found in all foods, with cereals and various organ meats being the richest sources.

Vitamin C

Chapter 8 told the story of Crandon's experiment with a vitamin C deficiency, as well as the sailors' problems with scurvy. Now let's pull the various functions of this very important vitamin together so that the full significance of this nutrient can be appreciated. From Crandon's work we know that vitamin C is necessary for the formation of the connective tissue, collagen. A deficiency during the period when teeth are forming can prevent calcification of the dentin, resulting in weak teeth that are more likely to be damaged than those with properly calcified dentin. This vitamin is also helpful in the absorption of iron and calcium from the intestinal tract, the conversion of folacin to its active form, and the metabolism of an amino acid, tyrosine.

Despite these varied and important functions for good health, not everyone in the United States is eating a diet that will provide the needed amount of the vitamin each day. Simply by being sure to eat a breakfast that includes a half cup of orange juice or a fresh orange, you can supply yourself with the needed quantity of vitamin C.

WATER

And with the few preceding comments about the water-soluble vitamins we shouldn't forget to add a few words about water. Water is part of nutrition, a very important part, and for several reasons. Water makes up about 60% of our total body mass. Water, via its evaporation from the lungs and skin is important and necessary in the regulation of body temperature. Water is necessary for the absorption and transport within the body of many nutrients and for the removal from the body of many waste products. Water also supplies some key mineral nutrients—calcium and magnesium, if the water is hard, occasionally iron and various trace minerals, and fluoride if you are lucky or live in a community that has the good sense to see that its water is fluoridated.

How much water each day? This is usually well regulated by various physiologic mechanisms, but for the average adult, somewhere around 6 to 8 glasses per 24 hours and this can be in the form of coffee, tea, milk, soft drinks, beer, etc. Fruits and vegetables are also good sources of water.

Need we write more about the importance of water? Yes, good water tastes good!

FIBER

Fiber is really not new in nutrition though it certainly has been given more attention recently. We used to refer to fiber as "roughage" or the non-digestible part of food that is important for providing bulk, absorbing water, and hence helping to form proper stools and avoid constipation. Fiber was given prominence a decade or so ago by two English physicians working in Kampala, Uganda. Drs. Trowell and Burkitt suggested that the reason most of their African patients had less disease of the bowel—cancer, diverticulitis, appendicitis, hemorrhoids, etc.—might be because they ate diets with far more fiber (roughage).

Our diets are low in fiber because they are based primarily on meat, milk, sugar, and white (refined) flour. The Ugandans had diets based on more vegetables and fruits, coarsely ground flour, and little meat and milk—hence more fiber.

As a result of the pioneering observations of Trowell and Burkitt much research has been done on fiber and fiber in foods. There are different types of fiber and they have different physiologic properties. It is easy to increase the fiber content of our diets—use more whole wheat breads, bran-containing cereals, more vegetables and fruits, and with the latter, more fruits of which we eat the skins like plums, grapes, and apples.

We think it desirable to increase the fiber content of our diets, but don't get the idea that fiber is a cure-all for all the diseases of mankind—it isn't. We do not approve of the big commercial push for bran—particularly unprocessed bran by the spoonful. It is wrong to suggest that bran and other types of fiber-containing foods will do anything for the "cholesterol problem." Hydrophilic "fiber" such as pectin and guar gum have some cholesterol-lowering effect, but it is small.

CONCLUSION

Nutrition is an important factor in good health. It is by no means the only factor—heredity, physical and mental activity, freedom from serious infectious diseases, an economic status to purchase the basics of health, are other factors important in good health. But one can write that good health is not possible without good nutrition.

With a modest understanding of nutrition, it is relatively simple to practice good nutrition. This consists of learning to eat and enjoy a variety of foods, a variety selected from among the Basic Four Food Groups, and of keeping total calorie intake over a period of a few days in balance with calorie output (physical activity), so that as a child proper growth and weight are obtained and as an adult proper weight is maintained.

We realize that a few of our nutrition colleagues do not like the Basic Four concept and prefer a return to the Basic Seven popularized during World War II. We disagree, in part probably because one of us (FJS) participated in originating the Basic Four concept, but particularly because we believe in simplification whenever possible. If one really eats a variety of fruits and of vegetables, one will come across citrus fruits and green and yellow vegetables to provide adequate vitamin C and A (carotene). That takes care of two of the Basic Seven Food Groups, and we feel there is enough fat in the American diet that a separate grouping of butter and margarine is unnecessary. So we are sticking to the Basic Four Food Groups and simply emphasizing variety within each of these four food groups.

As stressed in several places in this book, portion size is important and is the secret to calorie intake. It should be obvious that a 4-ounce steak has two-thirds the calories of a 6-ounce steak, and two cans of beer have twice the calories of a single can, and so on.

Muscular contraction by work or play requires energy and that energy comes from food in only four types—carbohydrate, fat, protein, or alcohol—by means of metabolic mechanisms that require various minerals, vitamins, and water. Contraction of muscles is the only way one has of using up calories, and in our experience most people, children or adults, who are obese are that way not because they consume huge amounts of calories but because they are inordinately inactive physically. They are people who after sitting six hours crossing the continent by air will use a moving sidewalk and an escalator to get out of the air terminal, who will wait five minutes for an elevator instead of walking two or three flights, who will take the car to visit friends who may live only a few blocks away, and so on ad infinitum.

Sugar has become a whipping boy for food faddists, consumer activitists, and we are sorry to write, a few nutritionists infatuated with the sound and sight of their names. But sugar in moderation has a useful role in most diets in that it is an efficient and less expensive source of calories, and one does need calories, particularly the active youngster and adolescent. And how much is moderation? Anywhere between 10 and 25 percent of our total calorie intake. These are the levels currently found in most of our diets as well as the diets of Europe.

Sugar is a constituent of many, many foods because the vast majority of the public enjoys its taste. It is thus partly responsible for these foods being eaten and their many nutrients obtained. A food that is not eaten and enjoyed, regardless of the nutrients it contains, is not contributing to better nutrition.

Food in the mouth is the cause of tooth decay, and there is very skimpy evidence that sugar consumed at mealtime increases tooth decay. There is to date only one practical way to lessen tooth decay and that is through the fluoridation of community water supplies. One can rant and rave about the so-called hazards of white refined sugar, about reducing sugar at mealtime, about fewer or no sweets in between meals, but one cannot "reform" people about sugar anymore than we could about alcohol. But in the real world we live in, tooth decay can be reduced 60 to 70 percent via fluoridation of community waters and another 10 to 15 percent by good dental care and newer dental techniques.

Finally, remember please, that so-called "health foods," organically grown foods, and natural foods are no more necessary for good nutrition than the green cheese of the moon which our astronauts did not find. Every food when properly used is a health food (even the red cherries in a Manhattan or old fashioned). Every food is an organic food and a fertile soil is filled with hundreds of organic and inorganic substances necessary for its development and growth. Every food is a natural food or made from natural sources.

So what to eat? Food, in variety from each of the Basic Four Food Groups. Food that you enjoy. Food from your favorite supermarket where you enjoy shopping. Don't eat too much; remember portion size. And insist that your local government get into the last half of the 20th century and adjust the fluoride content of your community water.

> This chapter brings us to the end of our book,
> At practical nutrition we took a close look,
> With all these suggestions on what you should eat,
> We wish you good health from food that's a treat!

RECOMMENDED BOOKS

NORMAL NUTRITION

FOOD AND FITNESS, Blue Cross Assoc., 840 N. Lake Shore Drive, Chicago, IL.

Guthrie, H. INTRODUCTORY NUTRITION, 4th ed., The C.V. Mosby Co., 1979.

Stare, F. and Aronson, V. DEAR DR. STARE, WHAT SHOULD I EAT? G. Stickley Co., 1982.

Stare, F. and McWilliams, M. LIVING NUTRITION, 3rd ed., John Wiley & Sons, 1980.

Stare, F. and Whelan, E. EAT OK—FEEL OK, Christopher Publishing House, 1978.

McGill, M. and Pye, O. THE NO NONSENSE GUIDE TO FOOD AND NUTRITION, Butterick Publishing, 1978.

INFANT AND CHILD CARE

Lambert-Lagace L. FEEDING YOUR CHILD, Collier-Macmillan Canada, Ltd., 1976.

McWilliams, M. NUTRITION FOR THE GROWING YEARS, 3rd ed., John Wiley & Sons, 1980.

TEENAGERS

Ikeda, J. FOR TEENAGERS ONLY, CHANGE YOUR HABITS TO CHANGE YOUR SHAPE, Bull Publishing Co., 1979.

Smith, N. HANDBOOK FOR THE YOUNG ATHLETE, Bull Publishing Co., 1978.

MATURE YEARS

Klinger, J. MEALTIME MANUAL FOR PEOPLE WITH DISABILITIES AND THE AGING, Mealtime Manual, Box 38, Ronks, PA, 1978.

EATING RIGHT FOR LESS, Consumer's Union, 1975.

FOOD FADS AND FACTS

Barrett, S. THE HEALTH ROBBERS, 2nd ed., G. Stickley Co., 1980.

Consumer Reports Books, Eds. HEALTH QUACKERY, Consumer's Union, 1980.

Deutsch, R. THE NEW NUTS AMONG THE BERRIES, Bull Publishing Co., 1977.

Stare, F. and Whelan E. PANIC IN THE PANTRY—FOOD FACTS, FADS, & FALLACIES, Atheneum, 1975.

Herbert, V. NUTRITION CULTISM—FACTS AND FICTIONS, G. Stickley Co., 1980.

Herbert, V. and Barrett, S. VITAMINS AND HEALTH FOODS—THE GREAT AMERICAN HUSTLE, G. Stickley Co., 1981.

WEIGHT CONTROL

Ferguson, J. HABITS NOT DIETS, Bull Publishing Co., 1976.
Simmons, R. THE NEVER SAY DIET BOOK, Warner Books, 1980.
Stuart, R. and Davis, B. SLIM CHANCE IN A FAT WORLD, Research Press Co., 1978.

HEART AND CIRCULATORY DISEASE

Eshleman, F. and Winston, M. THE AMERICAN HEART ASSOCIATION COOK-BOOK, 3rd ed., David McKay Co., 1979.
Margie, J. and Hunt, J. LIVING WITH HIGH BLOOD PRESSURE—THE HYPER-TENSION DIET COOKBOOK, HLS Press, Inc., 1455 Broad St., Bloomfield, NJ, 1978.

DIABETES

Gormican, A. CONTROLLING DIABETES WITH DIET, 2nd ed., Charles C Thomas, 1976.
Middletone, K. and Hess, M. THE ART OF COOKING FOR THE DIABETIC, Contemporary Books, 1978.
The American Diabetes Assoc. and The American Dietetic Assoc. THE FAMILY COOKBOOK, Prentice-Hall, Inc., 1980.

SELECTED TOPICS

Aronson, V. and Fitzgerald, B. GUIDEBOOK FOR NUTRITION COUNSELORS, Christopher Publishing House, 1980.
Bradley, H. and Sundberg, C. KEEPING FOODS SAFE, Doubleday and Co., 1975.
Clark, N. THE ATHLETE'S KITCHEN, CBI Publishing Co., 1981.
Kienholz, E. PET NUTRITION, Interstate Printers and Publishers, 1977.
Robertson, L., Flinders, C. and Godfrey, B. LAUREL'S KITCHEN: A HANDBOOK FOR VEGETARIAN COOKERY AND NUTRITION, Nilgiri Press, 1976.
Stern, J. S. and Denenberg, R. V. THE FAST FOOD DIET, Prentice-Hall, Inc., 1980.
Barrett, S. and Rovin, S. THE TOOTH ROBBERS: A PRO-FLUORIDATION HAND-BOOK, G. Stickley Co., 1980.
Cunningham, J. CONTROVERSIES IN CLINICAL NUTRITION, G. Stickley Co., 1980.

BOOKS ON NUTRITION—NOT RECOMMENDED

Airola, Paavo. (any book).
*Atkins, Robert. (any book).
Bassler, T. and Burger, R. The Whole Life Diet, M.E. Evans and Co., 1979.
*Bieler, H. Food is Your Best Medicine, Random House, 1965.
*Cheraskin, Emanuel. (any book).
Clark, Linda. (any book).
*Cooper, J. Dr. Cooper's Fabulous Fructose Diet, M.E. Evans and Co., 1979.

Davis, Adelle. (any book).

Dufty, W. Sugar Blues, Chilton Book Co., 1975.

*Edelstein, Barbara. (any book).

*Feingold, Benjamin. (any book).

Fredericks, Carlton. (any book).

Hall, R. Food for Nought—The Decline in Nutrition, Harper and Row, 1974.

Hauser, Gayelord. (any book).

Hausman, P. Jack Sprat's Legacy, Richard Merkek Publishers, 1981.

Hightower, S. Eat Your Heart Out—How Food Profiteers Victimize the Consumer, Random House, 1976.

Hunter, Beatrice Trum. (any book).

Jacobson, Michael. (any book).

*Jarvis, D.C. (any book).

Kordel, Lelord. (any book).

Lappe, R. Diet for a Small Planet, Friends of the Earth/Ballentine, 1971.

Lasky, M. The Complete Junk Food Book, McGraw-Hill Book Co., 1977.

Linn, R. The Last Chance Diet, Bantam Books, 1977.

Llewellyn-Jones, D. Every Body. A Nutritional Guide to Life, Oxford Univ. Press, 1980.

*Martin, C. Low Blood Sugar—The Hidden Menace of Hypoglycemia, ARC Books, Inc., 1970.

Mazel, J. The Beverly Hills Diet, Macmillan Publishing Co., 1981.

Mindell, E. Vitamin Bible, Warner Books, 1979.

Myerson, B. and Adler, B. The I Love New York Diet, Morrow, 1982.

*Newbold, H. Mega-Nutrients for your Nerves, Berkley Publishing Co., 1978.

*Nittler, A. A New Breed of Doctor, Pyramid House, 1972.

Null, Gary. (any book).

Nutrition Search, Inc. Nutrition Almanac, McGraw-Hill Book Co., 1975.

Nyoti, S. You Are All Sanpaku, University Books, Inc., 1965.

Ohsawa, G. Zen Macrobiotics—The Art of Longevity & Rejuvenation, Ignoramus Press, 1966.

Pritikin, N. (any book).

Rodale Press. (any book or Prevention Magazine).

*Reuben, David. (any book).

*Shute, E. and Taub, H. Vitamin E for Ailing and Healthy Hearts, Pyramid House, 1969.

*Stillman, I. and Baker, S. (any book).

*Schwartz, G. Food Power, McGraw-Hill Co., 1979.

*Tarnower, H. and Baker, S. The Complete Scarsdale Medical Diet, Rawson Wade Publishers, 1979.

Twitchell, P. Herbs—The Magic Healers, Lancer, 1971.

Veret, J. and Carper, J. The Case Against Food Additives, Simon and Schuster, 1974.

Wade, Carlson. (any book).

Walczak, M. Nutrition—Applied Personality, International College of Applied Nutrition, 1974.

Weiner, M. The Way of the Skeptical Nutritionist, Macmillan Publishing Co., 1981.

West, Ruth. (any book).

Whitmoyer, C. Your Health is What You Make It. Exposition Press, 1972.
Winter, Ruth. (any book).
*Yudkin, J. Sweet and Dangerous, Wyden Books, 1972.

*Unfortunately, these authors are M.D.'s.

SOURCES OF NUTRITION EDUCATIONAL MATERIALS

1. *Colleges and Universities*—Depts. of Home Economics, Nutrition, and Health Sciences.
2. *Food Industries*—Depts. of Home Economics, Consumer Relations, and Public Relations.
3. *Foundations Supporting Nutrition Education:*
   Nutrition Foundation, Inc., 887 17th Street, N.W., Washington, D.C. 20006.
4. *Government Agencies:*
   Food and Drug Administration, 5600 Fishers Lane, Rockville, MD 20857
   Food and Nutrition Information and Education Resources Center, National Agricultural Library, Room 304, 10301 Baltimore Blvd., Beltsville, MD 20705
   National Institutes of Health, Nutrition Coordinating Committee, Bethesda, MD 20205
   Superintendent of Documents, U.S. Government Printing Office, Pueblo, CO 81009
   Also, State and Local Health Departments.
5. *National Professional Organizations:*
   American Medical Association, Dept. of Food and Nutrition, 535 North Dearborn St., Chicago, IL 60610
   American Dietetic Association, 430 North Michigan Ave., Chicago, IL 60611
   American Geriatrics Society, 10 Columbus Circle, New York, NY 10019
   Society for Nutrition Education, 2140 Shattuck Ave., Berkeley, CA 94704
6. *Trade Associations:*
   Cereal Institute, 1111 Plaza Drive, Schaumberg, IL 60195
   National Dairy Council, 6300 North River Road, Rosemont, IL 60018
7. *Voluntary Health Organizations (National and Local Chapters):*
   American Heart Association, 7370 Greenville Ave., Dallas, TX 75231
   Arthritis Foundation, 3400 Peachtree Rd., Atlanta, GA 30326

INDEX

DATE DUE

AUG 3 1 1988		
DEC 1 4 1989		
4-30-90		
NOV 2 4 1997		

GAYLORD   PRINTED IN U.S.A.